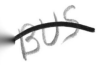

# Caring for People With Physical Impairment

## The Journey Back

Committee on Handicaps
Group for the Advancement of Psychiatry

William H. Sack, Portland, OR, *Chairperson*
Norman R. Bernstein, Cambridge, MA
Meyer S. Gunther, Wilmette, IL
Bryan King, Los Angeles, CA
Robert Nesheim, Duluth, MN
Betty J. Pfefferbaum, Norman, OK
William A. Sonis, Philadelphia, PA
Margaret L. Stuber, Los Angeles, CA
Thomas G. Webster, Washington, DC
Henry H. Work, Bethesda, MD

James R. Dumerauf, Waukesha, WI *(GAP Fellow)*

# Caring for People With Physical Impairment

## The Journey Back

Formulated by the
Committee on Handicaps

Group for the Advancement of Psychiatry

Report No. 135

Published by

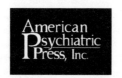

American Psychiatric Press, Inc.

Washington, DC
London, England

Copyright © 1993   Group for the Advancement of Psychiatry
ALL RIGHTS RESERVED
Manufactured in the United States of America on acid-free paper
96  95  94  93    4  3  2  1
Published by American Psychiatric Press, Inc.
1400 K Street, N.W., Washington, DC 20005

**Library of Congress Cataloging-in-Publication Data**

Caring for people with physical impairment  :  the journey back  /  formulated
    by the Committee on Handicaps, Group for the Advancement of Psychiatry.
        p.    cm. — (GAP report  :  no. 135)
    Includes bibliographical references and index.
    ISBN 0-87318-203-0
    1. Physically handicapped—Rehabilitation—Psychological aspects.
    2. Physically handicapped—Mental health. 3. Caregivers—Mental health.
    4. Medical personnel and patient. 5. Therapist and patient. I. Group for the
    Advancement of Psychiatry. Committee on Handicaps. II. Series: Report
    (Group for the Advancement of Psychiatry  :  1984)  ;  no. 135.
        [DNLM: 1. Caregivers. 2. Handicapped. 3. Rehabilitation. W1 RE209BR
    no. 135   /   WB 320 C277]
    RC321.G7 no. 135
    [RC451.4.H35]
    616.89 s—dc20
    [155.9′16]
    DNLM/DLC                                                              92-22055
    for Library of Congress                                                  CIP

**British Library Cataloguing in Publication Data**

A CIP record is available from the British Library.

The poems in this volume are used with permission as follows: Harold Bond
"The Game" (1970), from *Dancing on Water*, with permission of The Cummington
Press; Philip Dacey "The Handicapped," from *Night Shift at the Crucifix Factory*
(University of Iowa Press 1991), with permission of the author; Maxine Kumin
"Rehabilitation Center" (1961), from *The Nightmare Factory*, with permission of
Curtis Brown, Ltd.; Robert Phillips "The Persistence of Memory, the Failure of
Poetry" from *Personal Accounts* (Ontario Review Press 1986), with permission of
the Ontario Review Press; Anne Sexton "Doctors," from *Awful Rowing Toward
God* (Houghton Mifflin 1975), Copyright © 1975, Loring Conant, Jr., Executor of
the Estate of Anne Sexton, with permission of Houghton Mifflin, Co.; Ronald
Wallace "After Being Paralyzed From the Neck Down for Twenty Years," from
*Plums, Stones, Kisses and Hooks* (University of Missouri Press 1981), Copyright © 1981,
Ronald Wallace, with permission of the University of Missouri Press; Gary
Young "The Doctor Rebuilds a Hand" (1979), with permission of *Antaeus*/The
Ecco Press.

To George Tarjan, M.D., renowned psychiatric leader and friend, whose lifelong commitment to the care of all with physical and mental impairments was the guiding force in this work.

# Contents

## SECTION 1: BASIC CONCEPTS

## SECTION 2: CLINICAL APPLICATIONS

# SECTION 3: EDUCATIONAL APPLICATIONS

# Preface

The emergence of rehabilitation in the last several decades has helped meet the needs of several burgeoning populations who previously had been treated in ways that varied from neglectful to vile. Persons with disabilities, chronically ill individuals, elderly individuals—all have benefited by the development of rehabilitation teams and the promulgation of their basic tenets.

Physiatrists and their associates have been responsible for making collaborative medicine a bedside reality. By collaborative medicine I mean patient care that is integrated, multidisciplinary, and comprehensive. Such care requires a complex set of interactions among caregivers themselves, as well as interactions with the patient. Physiatry has applied with a flexible pragmatism an increasing number of scientific principles that include these interactive aspects.

Of these principles, none have been more essential than those embedded in dynamic psychiatry. At our hospital, the Rehabilitation Institute of Chicago, there is no person who has attended more to determining what these should be and ensuring that they are made usable and applicable than our psychiatrist, Meyer S. Gunther, one of the authors of this monograph. In the complexity of our interdisciplinary work, Dr. Gunther has struggled to show us how to keep the focus of effort on the individuality of the patient, demanding that each patient's team members ally with one another in their work toward common goals, ensuring that the patient gets the most intense, sensitive, and humane professional care possible. Our institution has richly benefited from the application of this psychological dimension into treatment.

If a staff member is to understand the feelings and attitudes of a patient, it is essential to also understand his or her own feelings. From insights into both one's self and one's patients, one can achieve the maximum in understanding the psychodynamics of rehabilitation and, as well, the ultimate in indirect satisfaction by working side by side with other staff struggling with the same issues.

There must be empathic participation on the part of *all* employees of a rehabilitation hospital. In this report, the authors show how experienced psychiatrists, using personal and professional skills, and working in a small-group educational format, can elevate staff psychological insights and abilities and then help staff to apply these insights in dealing with the physically impaired patient.

This report provides *concrete* guidelines to reach the goal of achieving staff self-awareness and, thus, the ability for productive action and participation. We at the Rehabilitation Institute of Chicago have been served well for 30 years by these concepts. They should help all caregivers to achieve the following:

1.  To provide the maximally effective therapeutic milieu for each patient.
2.  To analyze the components that are necessary to establish such a concept.
3.  To highlight that the psychological needs of the patients must always be kept in the forefront.
4.  To stress that all staff must learn to develop interpersonal skills in order to be able to cope with the complex psychodynamics of rehabilitation care.
5.  To recognize the vital role that staff self-knowledge and self-awareness have in bringing all this about.

Over the entrance to the Oracle of Delphi there was only one "simple" phrase, "Know thyself."

For those caregivers working with persons with physical impairments, this simple phrase represents a cogent motif. This achievement is not a simple matter for most organizations. This report sets practical goals and excellent guidelines on how to bring about such a total therapeutic approach. Those of us in rehabilitation medicine owe a debt of gratitude for the authors' contribution to such a significant component of our mission.

Henry B. Betts, M.D.
*Medical Director and Chief Executive Officer*
*Rehabilitation Institute of Chicago*
*Chicago, Illinois*

# Acknowledgments

We acknowledge here individuals who provided valuable assistance to members of the Committee on Handicaps of the Group for the Advancement of Psychiatry. Assisting from their perspective as physiatrists were Elliot Roth, M.D., Nancy Ball, M.D., and Matthew Eckmann, M.D. Harlan Hahn, Ph.D., provided valuable input on the community issues chapter. Robert Russ provided exceptional insights on the experience of having a physical disability. Robert Polland, Director of Camping Services of the Courage Center in Minneapolis, gave the committee a great deal of valuable consultation. Verena Michels, a social worker, and Sally McDermott, a hospital coordinator of volunteer services, also provided important input to the committee.

Finally, Ms. Judith Downs prepared the many versions of this manuscript with endless patience and good will.

# SECTION 1:
# BASIC CONCEPTS

## The Handicapped

**1**
The missing legs
Of the amputee
Are away somewhere
Winning a secret race.

**2**
The blind man has always stood
Before an enormous blackboard,
Waiting for the first
Scrawl of light,
That fine
Dusty chalk.

**3**
Here
The repetitions of the stutterer,
There
The flickering of the stars.

**4**
Master of illusion,
The paralytic alone moves.
All else is still.

**5**
At Creation,
God told the deaf,
"Only you will hear
The song of the stone."

**6**
Dare not ask
What the dumb
Have been told to keep secret.

**7**
When the epileptic
Falls in a fit,
He is ascending
To the heaven of earth.

*Philip Dacey*

# 1

# Introduction: A Rationale

Much has been written about the experience of having a physical impairment, both from the patient's and from the family's point of view. A good deal of professional writing has been directed to psychological specialists within the field of physical medicine and rehabilitation. But very little has been written for the nonspecialist caregiver who usually has the closest contact with the patient recovering from serious life-altering, appearance-altering bodily injury or congenital physical impairment. This monograph is an attempt to remedy such a situation.

The Committee on Handicaps of the Group for the Advancement of Psychiatry is a group of general and child/adolescent psychiatrists with considerable collective experience as consultants in hospitals, clinics, rehabilitation centers, and schools. Gathered from all parts of the United States, our committee meets twice a year to share experience and points of view in small-group discussion. The work in this monograph evolved over a 6-year span of time as we reviewed the current literature in the field and applied it to our particular experience.

Caregivers in all settings have strong feelings about their work and the patients for whom they care. Our consultation-liaison activity in rehabilitation settings has as frequently involved working with the feelings of caregivers as it has working with the problems of patients. The very nature of rehabilitation work carries with it the possibility for enormous personal fulfillment as well as sustained stress and burnout. Thus the experience of caregivers, even if overlooked in the literature, has importance as each patient makes the journey back with caregiving assistance.

## Why Now?

The need for such a volume as this seemed predicated on the very success of physiatry itself. (See Chapter 2 for a more full explanation of the history and current trends on the specialty of physical medicine and rehabilitation.) This field has enjoyed the application of ever more technological advances and procedures. Many individuals who suffered severe life-threatening physical impairment who would not have survived their injuries a generation ago are now living productive lives. Children with congenital anomalies are now leading useful lives in the community, whereas in the past they were often thought to be nonfunctional.

Physical medicine has now gained a secure position in many community hospitals, not only in technology but in service application. Moreover, the integration of psychosocial concepts into the treatment plans for patients is now also standard procedure. Mental health professionals are frequently an integral part of any rehabilitation team. Physiatry has grown not only in technological but in psychological sophistication.

Such sophistication brings in its wake increasing complexity, specialization, and a hierarchical framework of care. The talents of multiple caregivers of varying backgrounds must be integrated in order to carry out comprehensive care plans. Caregivers must work together in teams, usually led by a physician. The very hierarchy of care implies that those with the most technical skills and specialized backgrounds will be, of necessity, most removed from routine care tasks and moment-to-moment encounters with the physically impaired patient. (This includes the consulting psychiatrist as well.) The result is that while the overall care is organized by highly skilled professionals, the caregivers whom patients see and with whom they interact most frequently are the less specialized (but not less talented) professionals. These professionals "at the bedside" translate the care plan into a series of interpersonal-teaching transactions that have great meaning for both patients and their caregivers. Yet the psychological and psychosocial literature in physical rehabilitation is usually directed to the specialists and is often discipline-specific. A volume directed to more general providers of care—those actually physically closest to the recovering patient—would seem overdue. In this monograph we provide a psychosocial discussion applicable to caregivers who are both relatively new and less tied to a specific discipline.

This monograph is directed not only to the individual caregiver working at the bedside but also to nurses; nurses aides; physical, recreational, and occupational therapists; social workers and pastoral counselors; speech therapists; volunteers; and rehabilitation staff of diverse backgrounds and interests. While we hope that physiatrists might find useful information within these pages, the focus remains the nonphysician. Mental health professionals who have not had a great deal of prior clinical experience in this area may also find useful information here.

This monograph, *Caring for People With Physical Impairment: The Journey Back,* is so named because the process of rehabilitation can be viewed as an odyssey in which a variety of caregivers accompany each patient along part of this metaphorical journey. Such a journey implies a beginning, a middle, and then an ending, with the passage of time and a series of new experiences. Often the early setting of this journey for the patient with a severe physical impairment is in the hospital; then the journey continues, as the patient frequently moves to a rehabilitation center for weeks or months, followed by a return to home, family, and community (with concomitant contact with agencies, clinics, vocational training, and so forth).

Because caregivers can be seen as fellow travelers on part of this journey, the title of our work also implies a relationship that develops between patient and caregiver over time. It is this relationship of caregiving to a person with a physical impairment that occupies the central focus of this report. The basic investment of one person providing assistance to another transcends the particularities of disorder or the nature of the professional skill. While it is often true that the caregiver has traveled on this rehabilitation journey with others before and thus often functions as a "guide," the gigantic unknowns for the patient through this whole process are frightening indeed. No two persons are exactly alike. Hence the "journey back" is unique for each person. It is not true, however, that the caregiver is providing the "fuel" for the journey while the patient passively "goes along for the ride." Such an assumption would go against most of the basic principles of rehabilitation medicine itself. Rather, in this journey both fellow travelers are active participants. Both share a set of specific goals, and both are using all their capacities to achieve these goals.

The rewards for the caregiver in making this "trip" can be substantial, and a later chapter (see Chapter 9) is devoted to spelling these rewards out in some detail. Helping to make another's life more useful has its own intrinsic satisfactions. All caregivers want this journey to be a success for each of their patients. But like any kind of travel, there are risks along the way, particularly when success for the caregiver means emotional investment in the patient and the process. What are some of these risks?

First, there is the risk of failure. The efforts caregivers expend may not result in the improvement they expect. The patient's sense of failure may have reverberations on the caregivers' self-esteem. Second, patients may not cooperate; they may oppose suggestions and insist on their own ideas. Caregivers and patients may come into conflict, with consequent frustration and anger in both. Third, caregivers may fear for the physical and emotional safety of those in their charge. As patients venture forth into a world that is not always benevolent or caring, caregivers cannot anticipate the pressures these patients will experience, nor can caregivers protect them from these pressures. Caregivers cannot protect them from the social isolation or loneliness of life in some community settings or from the stigma that befalls some patients. Fourth, concerns about the families of patients are ubiquitous. Will the families be up to the new burdens and responsibilities of care (not to mention the financial pressures)? Will they invest in this care as their hospital caregivers have done? Will current viewpoints on important aspects of daily care be shared by key family members?

Finally, investing in the care of persons with physical impairment means tolerating and sharing their feelings as they struggle to build or rebuild their lives. Being with the patient means feeling not only the pride in new gains, but the anger at the injustice over the impairment itself, the bitterness at what is lost and cannot be regained, the helplessness of a body now compromised, and the despair about a self whose worth is questioned and whose future is uncertain. Being to some extent a fellow traveler puts the caregiver in the position of sharing the same pain one wishes to overcome in the patient.

## Some Basic Premises

The reader will soon notice the heavy emphasis given to subjective experience in this work. So much of physical medicine's clinical success is described in "objective" terms (e.g., range of limb movement, percentage return of function, etc.), as it should be. Yet behind the objective improvement lies a large and rich subjective experience—full of the joys and sorrows of not only the physically impaired patient but the caregiver as well. Our fundamental premises are as follows:

1.  The caregiver needs to be ready to experience the subjective world of the patient as the two work together.
2.  Frequently the kinds of feelings caregivers experience are a reflection of what the patient is also feeling.
3.  Caregivers need to recognize within themselves the kind of feelings patients generate in them.
4.  Caregivers need to learn to harness those feelings in order to appropriately respond in an empathic manner to their patients.

5. When this caregiving empathic transaction occurs successfully, the patient feels understood and is able to tap more inner motivational resources for the tasks of rehabilitation. Likewise, caregivers who feel they more fully understand what is making their patients "tick" gain, besides more effective professional work with patients, a sense of inner fulfillment that means job satisfaction, job longevity, and less job burnout.

Consulting work with experienced caregivers and their patients has shown us that ignoring this experiential dimension of care involves real risks: discouraged and lonely patients and/or overstressed and frustrated caregivers who may emotionally abandon (or subtly attack) the patients in their charge. The "journey back" is a subjectively intense experience for both patient and caregiver. Most every emotion known to humankind is experienced along the way.

## The Caregiver and the Committee

Psychiatrists are not on the front lines of the care of people who have suffered serious physical impairments. We do not directly change their dressings, construct their prostheses, or teach patients to regain basic self-help skills. When care is routine and things are going smoothly, we will seldom be present. Only when conflicts within the patient or between patient and caregiver occur do we appear on the scene. Thus, this notion of writing a volume about the experiences of caregiving may seem presumptive, if not audacious. What claim can we make that we will have something of value to say to our intended audience?

Our collective experience as consultants has brought us into sustained contact with some very talented, very experienced caregivers from a variety of backgrounds. They have been our instructors. Yet their wisdom rarely gets into print because they are too busy doing what they are trained to do—that is, providing care. We wish to remind the reader that the collective voice of the committee also includes the many voices of caregivers toward whom we owe an enormous debt of gratitude. Our intention is that the "we" in this document be their voice as much as ours.

## Acquired Impairment, Congenital Impairment

Not being able to walk means something quite different to a person who has never ambulated than it does to someone who has ambulated most of one's life (Featherstone 1980). No single volume can adequately cover all caregiving facets in such wide-ranging arenas of care. People with a variety of physical impairments, both congenital and acquired, live and work in many places we have not been. In the present volume we focus primarily on individuals suffering from acquired impairments because that is where our experience lies. No pretensions of covering the vast experience of caregivers who work with the individuals with congenital impairment can be made. However, occasional references are made throughout this work to those who have impairments from birth (Tarnow 1984).

## Definitions

The three terms *impairment, disability,* and *handicap* are not always used correctly. The most concise definition of *impairment* is any loss of psychological, physiological, or anatomic structure or function. Impairments may be permanent or temporary, and they may be present from birth or acquired adventitiously. *Disability* refers to the impact of impairment on the performance of activities commonly accepted as the basic elements of everyday living (i.e., walking, talking, negotiating transportation, dressing, feeding, bathing, etc.). Disability can be used when an impairment constitutes a hindrance to any of these activities of daily living. *Handicap* is a term that has come to represent the more profound effects of impairments and disabilities that involve the whole person. It is the sum of social and environmental disadvantages to the individual resulting from disease, impairment, or disability. In the child it is a state that retards, disturbs, or otherwise adversely affects normal growth, development, and adjustment to life. In adults a handicap constitutes a disadvantage for a given individual in that it limits or prevents the fulfillment of a role that is normal for that individual. Impairment is more objective and is expressed in terms of symptoms; handicap is more subjective and is expressed in terms of social role (Thomas 1982).

One can have a sizeable disability with little handicap or a mild disability with major handicap. Thus handicap may appear at all levels of illness severity. The prevention of a handicap requires different interventions from those needed to prevent disability.

The most dramatic example of this disparity between handicap and disability is the famous scientist Stephen Hawking. He is confined to a wheelchair by his severe amyotrophic lateral sclerosis (physical disability) but is a productive theoretical scientist whose influential theories about the origins of the universe are widely respected (lack of concomitant handicap).

While these terms have a clinical precision about them, they also carry a strong emotional connotation for those whom they are intended to describe. Most affected people prefer the term "disability" to "handicap," and they remind us, "I have a handicap, I am not a handicapped person!"

In this monograph, both the terms "disability" and "impairment" will be used, but, when possible, the term "impairment" is preferred because of its generic quality. Any term is treacherous because any word can acquire a pejorative connotation. People with physical impairments resent being defined by what they cannot do; they would prefer to be defined by what they can do. Whenever one refers to someone else with an impairment, it is best to use positive rather than negative terms. Examples are "He walks with crutches" versus "He cannot walk without crutches," or "She uses a wheelchair" rather than "She is confined to a wheelchair." Traditionally, physicians have been guilty of couching their descriptions in terms of basic pathology that often carries a negative connotation with repeated usage over time. Caregivers are cautioned to be sensitive to the meanings of the words used and vigilant in correcting unnecessary negativity.

Terms used also depend on what stage of rehabilitation or recovery an individual is in. In this monograph people with physical impairments inside a hospital or rehabilitation center will be referred to as patients. Those in the community will be referred to as people, persons, or individuals. The word "patient" has been chosen, even though we are aware that others prefer terms such as "client." The severity of the problems these people face and the protracted nature of their care more than justifies the use of the term "patient" in this monograph. Offering assistance to another entails the risk of making the latter feel inferior. This is a basic caregiver issue that will be repeatedly addressed throughout.

## Organization

This volume can be used in a number of ways. It will provide a deeper understanding of caregiver-patient interactions when read in its entirety. Section 1 introduces the basic intent of this effort and the basic psychological concepts on which caregiving activities rest. It also includes (in Chapter 3) a generic description of the psychological experiences of having a severe, life-threatening, body-altering, appearance-altering injury. In Chapter 3 we shift the focus from the caregiver-patient transaction to the experience of the patient with a physical impairment per se, in order to provide a more adequate framework for understanding the many different issues germane to the caregiver. Section 1 ends with a discussion of caregiver experience from a developmental perspective (see Chapter 4).

Section 2 is the core of this work. It contains the application of the basic concepts listed in Section 1 to the caregiver's experience with the patient or physically impaired person. Caregiver experience has been divided into reactions, coping strategies, therapeutic transactions, and satisfactions. The section focuses often on caregiver-patient transactions in a rehabilitation setting. But also included is a chapter on caregiving in the community (see Chapter 8).

Section 3 is intended to stand separately from the previous sections. The chapters in this section are presented as an educational guide for those who intend to use this volume in inservice training programs in hospitals, rehabilitation centers, and clinics. Vignettes are provided that raise particular management problems and challenge caregivers to examine their own reactions as they discuss potential solutions. This section also contains a chapter on psychiatric consultation in a rehabilitation setting, the intent of which is to acquaint non–mental health professionals with the particular roles and functions of the consultant.

The journey back from a physical impairment is for the patient a continuing re-creation of a new life from the pieces of the old. It is a process that requires sojourners who are able to assist in re-creating the new from the old. It is a necessity, for as John Hull (1991) writes about his experience of becoming blind, "One must re-create one's life or be destroyed" (p. 179).

Our hope is that this monograph can evoke an ongoing dialogue with our reader. Perhaps this discussion will then get renewed in other places (such as the coffee shop, team meeting, etc.) as caregivers participate with the patient in the journey of rehabilitation.

## A Question of Energy

I'm not diminished
    by this loss of limb
I'm more than
    the sum of my parts
to deny my scars
    is to deny my power
the core of heat in each cell.

I've got wires humming
    juices surging
        detours on the path
it takes less time now
less resistance
to complete the circuit
      I'm well grounded
          you can touch me
            without a shock.

*Amber Coverdale Sumrall*

2

# Conceptual Foundations

I n this chapter we summarize the clinical and psychological concepts used in constructing this report. Descriptions of these concepts are brief and may be somewhat oversimplified. However, more information can be readily obtained in the references listed.

Psychiatrists bring to any topic particular ways of understanding human behavior based on a number of underlying theories or constructs. Our committee has been richly influenced by a range of theorists who are psychodynamically oriented (Horowitz 1976; Kohut 1971, 1977; Winnicott 1958), systems oriented (Goffman 1961, 1963), or focused on stress and coping (Lazarus and Folkman 1984). Before attending to particular concepts in the psychological realm, we review briefly the history and pivotal position of rehabilitation medicine itself in the care of physically impaired individuals.

## The Basic Concept of Rehabilitation Medicine

In contrast to more traditional approaches to acute care and chronic diseases, rehabilitation medicine is characterized by several striking approaches that at first may appear paradoxical. Patients are stable (more or less), that is, no longer acutely ill but hardly cured. They are still relatively nonfunctional. The aim of rehabilitation is achievement of optimal functional capacity, but this hardly constitutes restoration to a state of pre-illness normalcy (which is impossible). Sometimes rehabilitative aims are achieved via compensatory mechanisms, such as prostheses. But the crucial approach in rehabilitation is everything biopsychosocial in relationship to everything else, and all at the same time. This may be likened to an encompassing *syncytial*, or merging, approach instead of a linear "one thing at a time" (the more usual biomedical) effort.

The rudiments of rehabilitation medicine and physiatry have been present in several medical specialties (e.g., orthopedics) since the 1920s. But rehabilitation medicine as a separate, integrated specialty grew out of the need to care for a large number of seriously impaired survivors in our society, the result of people living longer and of catastrophic world as well as local events, coupled with technical medical advances. For instance, following World War II the United States had thousands of severely physically impaired soldiers with a permanent residue of "incurable" orthopedic, neuromuscular, or special sensory defects. The goal of care was optimal adaptive capacity to function again in usual life roles—such as those involving self-care, mobility, and vocation, as well as social and family roles—rather than a "cure." New methods pioneered by such leaders of physical medicine and rehabilitation as Howard Rusk (1977) focused on optimal restoration via re-education or re-arrangement of existing capacities, discovery of unrecognized capacity, or substitution of mechanical assistive devices (orthoses) or whole-area replacement devices (prostheses) for impaired or lost functions. Optimal restoration also included a recognition of the crucial effects of cognitive and personality components of the impairment.

Over the past 40 years rehabilitation medicine has become a recognized specialty in the majority of American medical schools. The primary tools of rehabilitation remain technology, teaching, and therapy in a clinical setting that is individualized, empirical, flexible, and collaborative. The patient is an active participant in all levels in the process, not just the passive recipient of medical effort. Because multiple systems of the body are damaged, multiple specialties and specialists are needed, working together as an interdisciplinary team of collaborating experts. Integration of the work of such a varied group is vital; thus the physician in rehabilitation medicine is often as much an integrator/leader as a hands-on "doer." Interdisciplinary collaboration and teamwork, while useful in other specialties, are vital in rehabilitation. No one can labor long in this field without needing the assistance of other caregiver professionals. As much as a physically impaired person needs the assistance of a caregiver, caregivers need the cooperative assistance of each other.

These principles are stated clearly in DeLisa's (1988) textbook on rehabilitation medicine:

> Since rehabilitation is a holistic and comprehensive approach to medical care, the combined expertise of an interdisciplinary team is necessary. The team approach is critical to solve the complex problems. A "health care team" is defined as a group of health care professionals

from different disciplines who share common values and work toward common objectives . . . (p. 3)

A team is usually led by the physician in charge. Although other physicians interested in rehabilitation may lead the team, the physiatrist has special skills in the evaluation of neuromuscular, musculoskeletal, and cognitive systems. As the leader of the team, the physician has broad responsibilities in that he or she is the pilot of the combined medical treatment and rehabilitation programs. . . .

The traditional model in which the physician assumes an authoritarian role and other team members "obey" may function effectively in some medical settings but not on the rehabilitation team. In this setting every team member should be encouraged to develop leadership to perform the task necessary for meeting the patient goals. (p. 5)

The reader will note that these principles are not now the exclusive domain of rehabilitation medicine. Other physicians and health care professionals are guided by these working concepts as well. We shall have more to say about the interdisciplinary care team in Chapter 6.

As mentioned before, many of the ways that people recover from injury are described in objective terms (i.e., range of motion of an arm or leg, percentage of functional capacity, tasks of daily living, etc.). Caregivers in rehabilitation settings are under pressure to improve these objective measures to the greatest possible extent, because rehabilitation plans are always formed around goals based upon such objective measures.

Psychiatrists have long accepted the legitimacy of the subjective in all human experience. A primary aim in this monograph will be to highlight what is less visible and thus less measurable, but no less important in determining long-term outcome: the subjective interplay between patient and caregiver based on aroused or reactive intrapsychic factors of which neither participant is fully aware (Nussbaum 1984). It is this hidden dimension of reciprocal motivations that so often determines the experiential drama that gets played out in a variety of settings in which one person offers help to another (regardless of how the objective measures change). That is one reason why several of our chapters open with poetry—poetry being an expression of creative subjectivity.

We now present a summary sketch of several psychological concepts that have more specifically influenced our thinking about caregiving.

## The Body Image

The term *body image* (Schilder 1950) describes the nuclear, kinesthetic-tactile-visual sense of what we imagine we look like from the outside and what we feel like from the inside. It is highly individualistic, largely subjective, experienced as whole, integrated in space, and stable over time. As Jonathan Miller (1978) has said, "Our body is not, in short, something we have, it is a large part of what we actually are" (p. 14).

Everyone reacts emotionally when first viewing another's disfigured body. Painful reactions to another's disfigurement have their developmental roots in early, "forgotten" experiences of the first years of life. It is during those early months of existence that the infant learns to know himself or herself and significant others through perceptions of his or her own and others' bodies. As R. P. Burns (1975) states, "Learning about what is and what is not self, through direct experience and perception of the physical world[,] is the child's first step in the life journey, and the child sees body image and body schema as part of one's basic identity; which is then a major source of self-concept" (p. 150). In the infant's earliest perceptions, body and self are one. Discomfort or anxiety on initially experiencing another's disfigured body is developmental and ubiquitous; it is not necessarily neurotic or prejudicial.

Seeing another's malformed body threatens our own bodily integrity and self-image before we quite consciously recognize what has happened. We cannot overemphasize this point. New caregivers need to know that their strong and painful reactions to another's bodily defect are normal and to be expected. Kleck (1966) showed experimentally that subjects who interacted with physically disabled people reported more psychological discomfort as compared with their interactions with nonimpaired individuals. Caregivers need to be able to monitor their own subjective reactions to their patients in order to both obtain important information and give as appropriate responses as possible. Rather than avoiding anxiety by distancing themselves from a particular patient, caregivers need to examine their feelings and harness them in the service of optimal care. All good inservice training programs make explicit these issues.

## Boundary Issues

When someone is both acutely and badly injured, the boundaries of how one perceives oneself and others can get fuzzy and confused. Patients can develop fantasies and behaviors about how their caregivers should relate to them that can be grossly unrealistic and thus unsettling for those in their charge. The analogy we like best in explaining these expectations is "the genie in Aladdin's bottle"—that is, the expectation that the caregiver should always be at the beck and call of the patient. The implication is that the caregiver is not another autonomous person but only a representation of the patient's will and so should be at the total disposal of only the patient. This rather demanding attitude can also be coupled with patients' parallel expressions of the absolute indispensability of the caregiver. Such an interaction is bewildering indeed to a caregiver who has no prior experience to fall back on in such an encounter. The burden on any caregiver is formidable! With time, the acutely ill patient recognizes that a secure, dependable caregiver relationship is possible. Caregiving tasks then get easier. The danger for the caregiver is that he or she may not recognize the temporary aspect of this transaction. (This interaction will again be taken up in Chapter 5.)

Another foundational concept, *vulnerability*, refers to how terribly unprotected, helpless, easily frightened, and hurt the patient feels in the face of special burdens or losses, such as a catastrophic illness. Vulnerability particularly applies to feelings of potential or actual loss of one's self worth, value, or power as a human being. It is a very predictable, "normal" reaction to body damage. Expressions of such vulnerability might be undue anger at small irritations that one could ordinarily tolerate, or demands for special treatment and consideration. One can easily imagine how both "boundary" difficulties and vulnerability are intermixed in early phases of care:

> One of us was called to see an 81-year-old former executive who had suffered a stroke 1 week prior to the consultation. He was bitter and told one of the nurses he was going to "really do the job right" when he got home. It was difficult to understand just where this man's suicidal intent was coming from until he blurted out, "See, I can't even hold any urine anymore." Incontinence in the early stages of recovery can be a devastating loss, particularly to someone who has prided oneself on "control" of all kinds throughout one's life. This man's incontinence cleared over the next week as did his suicidal ideation.

A central psychological task of the victims of catastrophic illness is that of changing both their body image and the ambitions and values that are part of their personalities—a task mandated by the anatomic-physiological changes. To effect changes in both these structures is not a simple, conscious problem-solving task, as if the individual were simply to rearrange pieces of himself or herself on a sheet of paper until the pattern became more pleasing. The process is one of trial and error in which a good deal of inner reluctance must be overcome and considerable grieving over losses and changes undertaken. It involves concrete behavioral experiences in which one learns how one's body (and self) really are not the same as before. The physically impaired patient's life role capabilities have been significantly altered, and life's aims and activities must change accordingly. Such enormous psychological work takes time.

The neurologist Oliver Sacks (1984), at the time recovering from a serious leg injury, has described the indivisibility of body image and self-image thus:

> ... But what was now becoming frightfully, even luridly, clear was that whatever had happened was not just local, peripheral, superficial—the terrible silence, the forgetting, the inability to call or recall—this was radical, central, fundamental. What seemed at first, to be no more than a local peripheral breakage and breakdown now showed itself in a different, and quite terrible, light—as a breakdown of memory, of thinking, of will—not just a lesion in my muscle, but a lesion in me. The image of myself as a living ship—the stout timbers, the good sailors, the directing captain, myself—which had come so vividly to my mind in the morning, now re-presented itself in the lineaments of horror. It was not just that the good sailors were deaf, disobedient or missing, but that I, the captain, was no longer captain. I, the captain, was apparently brain damaged—suffering from severe defects, devastations, of memory, of thought. I fell very suddenly, and mercifully, into an almost swoon-like sleep. (p. 67)

Such life-altering illnesses usually leave evidence that makes it apparent to the world that something catastrophic has happened. Whether it is a scar, a prosthesis, or a wheelchair, there is an enormous impact upon one's altered sense of self and worth. Both the patient and the caregiver are inevitably affected by such bodily changes.

Along with these characteristics must be added the issue of new and uncertain experiences of time. Earlier assumptions about one's life are shattered. The future is imbued with uncertainty. The patient is now often more vulnerable to everyday physical or psychological stress, to intercurrent infections, and to the early onset of fatigue. A typical and highly constructive adaptation is to become "self-centered"—that is, self-protective, self-oriented, and self-concerned in order to husband one's resources. The patient may become quite selective about devoting any energy to the good of other persons under such new circumstances. As a result, some such persons with physical impairments are often accused of being "selfish." Such a reaction is common. The self-centeredness wanes as the patient improves, as in the following case:

> One of us caring for a seriously burned 6-year-old child was asked to provide consultation to the child's mother, who, also seriously burned, was on another ward of the same hospital. The request came from the nursing staff, who were concerned that this mother showed no apparent interest to the current life-threatening condition of her daughter. The consultant found that the mother was so involved in her own struggle for survival that she had no emotional resources for this added

psychological task. This knowledge immediately relieved the nurses' anxiety about the mother's nurturing capacity. Several weeks later the mother had improved physically and was anxious to see her daughter.

## A Transactional Relationship

People become neither catastrophically damaged nor rehabilitated in isolation. It is impossible to talk adequately about a physically impaired person's struggles without including the context of those struggles: relationships between patient and caregiver and between patient and family. This approach, the *transactional* view of human existence, has a long history: in the study of perceptions (Ittelson 1962); in developmental psychology (Sameroff and Chandler 1975); and in psychiatry (Grinker 1971). Emde's studies (Emde et al. 1986) of mother-child interactions have been particularly relevant to the transactions between the patient and the caregiver. The term *transactional* as used here refers to the many ways a patient's responses affect the caregiver and the ways that the caregiver's response affects the patient, so that both patient and caregiver are changed in and through this process. Such an interchange proceeds via an evolving series of stepwise reciprocal encounters.

Transactional processes of this kind have taken their place only recently in the history of scientific research. Before the 20th century, Newtonian physics assumed that the observer was outside the system being observed; an observation was taken to be independent of the observing process. Now the limitations of this view are realized. Physics has led the way to our appreciating that the act of observing influences what is observed (see, e.g., Bohr 1928; Heisenberg 1927). This principle is no less true for psychological science. We participate as we observe; we influence and are influenced by what we are observing (Emde et al. 1986).

Our task is not to hide these mutual influences but to make use of them in patient care. An infinite array of feelings in both participants flow from these mutual influences. We influence each other at all levels and dimensions. For example, we may respond to a physically disabled person's depression with depressive feelings of our own and then react in various ways to those feelings. Recognizing those feelings, we might respond with understanding, availability, and caring—that is, through some effort to overcome the sadness in both of us. In contrast, we may restrict our feelings, pull back, become removed, and even emotionally abandon the patient. Either way, a physically impaired person will then resonate to the caregiver's response, and the interactive process will continue at a new level. Transactional processes of this sort are familiar to all who have dealt with physically impaired adults, children, and their families. Yet, this dimension rarely gets much attention, let alone recognition for its great clinical value. It is easier (and more comfortable) to describe the physically disabled individual's struggles and leave out our own.

Why is it so difficult to accord this experience appropriate recognition? Patient and caregiver generate defenses to deal with many such potentially troublesome feelings; these defenses can then lead to a breakdown in the interactive process. In addition, the coping through which a physically impaired person moves from acute injury to a full rehabilitation has its "mirror" in the reciprocal struggles over coping in the caregiving staff. Both are part of a process that is as similar as it is different. Yet the responsive experience of the caregiver is often the shadowy, transactional "left hand" of the patient's rehabilitation process.

## Loss

The appreciation of loss is crucial for caregivers interacting with people who have body-altering, appearance-altering impairments (Hamburg and Adams 1967). Every individual who enters a physical rehabilitation program has experienced a significant, "unexpected" loss, and for many it is the most devastating loss of their lives. As David Krueger (1984) eloquently points out, "The disabled mourns the body, the function, the identity, the mobility, and the future aspiration that might have been" (p. 4). Experienced caregivers learn to anticipate a loss reaction in their patient at some point along the rehabilitation journey as the patient gradually feels the full impact of these losses. Adults missing a limb mourn for future aspects of the world lost to them because of their mutilation, as much as for the lost limb itself.

The same is true for a parent who gives birth to a child with a congenital deformity. A marked disequilibrium in the early parent-child relationship is often the case, as the parent grieves the loss of the hoped-for or expected child of fantasy. Slowly the new, actual impaired child is accepted in its place. This process takes both work and time on the part of each family member (Niederland 1965).

## The Family

The family members that stand beside the physically impaired patient during the rehabilitation process and to which the patient must return are crucially important. The family can reinforce or sabotage the best efforts of caregivers. Every alliance that is formed between the patient and the caregiver must also include the family (Krueger 1984). For the majority of patients, without their family's support virtually nothing permanent and useful will be obtained during rehabilitation.

During the crises of the discovery of a congenital impairment or immediately following an acute injury, families are vulnerable to confusion and disorganization. They may not hear or accept what is said to them, or they may confuse important medical information. Caregivers need to recognize that basic information may need to be repeated several times in order for it to "sink in"; for anxiety can momentarily cripple one's ability to retain and assimilate. It is helpful if one of the caregiving team can act as a family coordinator and liaison to family members so that the information they receive is both clear and consistent. For example, Maus-Clum and Ryan (1981) found that families of brain-injured patients almost unanimously rated "receiving a clear explanation" as their top priority of service need at the time of acute injury.

One of the major tasks of the caregiving team is to determine what coping strategies the patient and his family habitually utilize (i.e., before injury) and how these coping methods can now be harnessed to serve the patient's new challenge of physical and emotional rehabilitation (Krueger 1984). As rehabilitation proceeds, the family's ways of interacting with each other and the physically impaired family member need to be altered because traditional ways of relating may no longer work. Families must give up many of their old ways of interacting and mobilize their strengths to support and reintegrate the newly physically impaired member. At the same time, families must buffer the stresses and strains of changed roles and new activities on each member. This function should be made especially available as the newly received member ventures forth to test his or her capabilities and limitations at work or school.

Families engage in various defenses that are similar to the defenses patients themselves use (see Chapter 3). The family may attempt to minimize or deny the seriousness of the injury at first. Later, they may "bargain" with caregivers by assuming that their full involvement in care will magically bring full restorative or cure to their damaged family member. They, too, must grieve and work through their loss feelings as rehabilitation proceeds. Finally, over time their accommodation to the disability frees their energies for the tasks at hand (Bray 1987).

## Empathy

Empathy is a core concept on which depends much of one's understanding of any troubled individual. Our understanding of this concept comes primarily from the psychotherapy literature, most recently explicated and popularized by the self-psychology school (e.g., Basch 1980, 1988;

Book 1988). The first of its two primary meanings refers to empathy as a data-gathering technique.

One may gather vital subjective data about another person's conscious and unconscious emotional states by imaginatively attempting to stand within the experiencing self of the patient. At the same time that one is participating selectively with the patient, one is observing one's own participation in this state of the patient. It is this dual, constantly shifting subjective/objective process that distinguishes *empathy* from identification (and from projection), where one loses objectivity and a conscious sense of the interaction (Book 1988).[1] Empathy thus reflects the subjective experience of the caregiver through which he or she affectively and cognitively comprehends the inner experience of the patient. At its highest level, empathic comprehension focuses on understanding the total meaning of the patient's experience in the patient's own terms. Thus, empathic comprehension has the potential to lead to genuinely empathic responses.

This introduces the second meaning of empathy: an attitude of benevolent helpfulness; a selectively tuned concern for the other; a willingness to "stand alongside" the patient, valuing the patient as a person and accepting the legitimacy of the patient's feelings and ideas whatever they may be. To understand the other in his or her "total" terms becomes the first phase of offering authentic assistance to our patients. Professionals working in rehabilitation settings are justifiably skeptical of "do gooders" who tend to infantilize patients or indulge them toward regression. Thus, we wish to make a sharp distinction between empathy (or an empathic approach) and simple goodwill, kindness, or sympathy. A short case example may help:

> One of us, consulting in a military hospital, watched a singular interaction between a severely facially burned corporal and his nurse. The nurse, with a touch of sarcastic humor, referred to this man as "dog face." After the consultant got over his initial shock and watched further interactions between patient and nurse, he noticed a good deal of respect and closeness. It seemed that when the nurse addressed this man in such a superficially "derogatory" way, she was really also

---

[1]By *identification* we mean the unconscious taking in of qualities or characteristics, originally acquired by imitation, of someone who is emotionally important to us (either admired or feared). By contrast, *projection* is a mental mechanism by which an unwelcome idea or threatening feelings are disguised by being regarded as belonging to the external world or to someone else (i.e., pushed out of one's own mind and attributed to some else's).

saying, "You are a tough soldier who has been through a lot. You have a facial injury, but you are also a potentially normal soldier who knows how to take it. I will assume you continue to have these qualities. I will also acknowledge your facial scars directly, the way others might someday do."

Granted, this reflection on the consultant's part was pure speculation, yet we felt that this blunt response on the nurse's part contained within it a good deal of empathy and understanding. Her "free" expression might have moved this soldier closer to accepting his facial disfigurement. Sometimes, it is as important *how* something is said as the words themselves. There are no formulas or rules that easily apply. Caregivers cannot be too categorical.

As this chapter closes, we offer one vignette in which empathic understanding was crucial in resolving a psychological crisis:

> One of us was called to a rehabilitation ward to see an acutely agitated adolescent paraplegic male who was threatening suicide. He had broken a glass and had the jagged edge poised against his wrist as he angrily swore at the staff for what he considered their controlling tactics. The consultant came in, sat down, and said, "Jim, if I'd been through what you've been through, I might feel like killing myself, too. Maybe death is the best solution. But for a moment let's look and see if maybe there aren't other ways to handle some of your problems. If these don't work, you are always free later to try suicide. But for now, let's look for some other things." Jim dropped the glass and began to cry. The consultant was then able to conduct a productive interview.

This open acknowledgment that Jim's suicidal ideas had a legitimacy was the initial step in helping the young man feel "understood." Empathy with Jim's desperate plight allowed the consultant to respond effectively in a manner typical of what Winnicott would call "holding" or Kohut would call "empathic merging."

## The Persistence of Memory,
## The Failure of Poetry

The severed hand flutters
     on the subway track,
like a moth. No—
it is what it is,
     *a severed hand.*
It knows what it is.
And all the king's doctors
     and all the king's surgeons
put hand and stump together
again. Fingers move,
     somewhat. Blood circulates,
somewhat. "A miracle!" reporters
     report. But it will only
scratch and claw, a mouse
     behind the bedroom wall. We forget.
At four a.m. the hand
     remembers: intricate musical
fingerings, the metallic
feel of the silver flute.

*Robert Phillips*

3

# The Experience of
# Physical Impairment

While this volume primarily focuses on the subjective experiences of caregivers, we momentarily shift that focus in this chapter to trace the psychological reactions of people who have sustained life-altering physical impairments and are beginning their "journey back" through the experiences of rehabilitation. Our discussion of patient responses will be presented in terms of sequential stages for the purpose of simplicity, acknowledging that these stages are an artificial abstraction and that any particular reaction may be seen at any one time. These generalizations are a product of a review of the rehabilitation literature, as well as the committee's observations. Although different illnesses pose somewhat different behavioral and psychological threats, it is the basic similarities in how people cope with life-threatening, life-altering, body-function–altering, or appearance-altering catastrophic impairments and their often ignored meaning that shall be the focus of this chapter.

## Traumatic Disorganization

Any individual's initial focus after sustaining physical impairment is on dealing with the discomfort, incapacity, and symptoms associated with the bodily damage itself. There may be a certain numbness and disbelief connected with the experience, coupled with a vague sense of threat or self-blame. Constriction of interests and mild cognitive disorganization, often in the form of persistent confusion about what is happening, can lead to a withdrawal and turning inward to a more self-protected,

self-concerned orientation, with temporary loss of investment in interpersonal relationships. The predominant feelings that accompany this
initial state are anxiety (including, at times, overt fright), irritation
(sometimes to the point of outright rage), and a feeling of utter aloneness
or estrangement from one's body, termed *depersonalization*. Such trau-
matically induced psychological disorganization, followed by adaptive
regression, reduces the patient's world to a focus on the body and its
care. Thus dependency on others is generally welcomed by the patient
in this initial phase. Such a stage usually lasts only a few days.

## Initial Stabilization

This dependency on others generally (temporarily) develops into a
wish-based belief that compliance with caregivers will result in restoration of function, a belief often covertly encouraged by the caregivers. The
patient becomes passive, cooperative, and somewhat childlike, in the
trust that this is what is required for recovery. A false pleasantness hides
underlying depressed feelings, and relationships with caregivers take
on a superficial idealization. This may be a pleasant time for patient and
caregiver, although both recognize at some level how deceptive this
initial adjustment really is. Nothing has yet been confronted, struggled
with, or sorted through to some preliminary state of resolution. Yet, this
early period of stabilization serves a crucial function in that it permits
the individual a brief respite from confrontation with the full implications of the impairment. Denial is appropriately used temporarily
to allow the individual time to adapt to the injury and to set the stage
for rehabilitation. Denial can then be gently confronted and the patient
helped to move on to a more active coping approach, as the following
case illustrates:

> A 10-year-old girl who had recently undergone an amputation of her
> leg at the hip because of a malignancy vigorously fought any and all
> attempts to introduce a prosthesis. She would have nothing to do with
> any discussion of her rehabilitation. In talking with the girl, it became
> clear that she believed, if she waited, "my leg will grow back again."
> Not psychotic, this girl clung to the common but magical notion of
> restoration by passivity. A psychiatric consultant helped her work
> through the permanence of her loss, and in several days she accepted
> her new prosthesis.

The duration of this stage is highly variable but can last for several
weeks.

## The Second Crisis: Disorganization, Regression, and Confrontation With Basic Issues

Also called the period of depression, the term "second crisis" more adequately conveys the degree of turmoil often encountered clinically during this phase. It is a time of intense psychological pain for the patient and maximal stress for those attending the patient. As the patient regains some equilibrium and begins to be faced directly with everyday self-help activities and regular social activities, the previous denial and magical hopes of the initial stabilization must give way to the sobering reality of new limitations. Denial is not a conscious mental process. Thus caregivers cannot expect to discuss this issue with the patient. Yet it is crucial that caregivers recognize and respect this self-protective mechanism.

One can see how important early denial is for the patient. It helps titrate the recognition of the full extent of the injury to a reasonably tolerable degree. As the patient confronts the severity of the damage and its associated loss of function, the feelings of terror, helplessness, and grief may be very strong. Also mourned is the loss of imagined invulnerability or immortality, unconsciously held by most individuals well into adult life. If the patient is in a supportive environment, these reactions can be ameliorated somewhat but cannot be removed. However, most patients recognize that life will go on in spite of a change in anatomy, function, or appearance. This gradual realization allows the patient to begin facing up to the actual physical dilemmas and to prepare for the struggle to gain a "new" life. Confronting, accepting, and working through the feelings is a slow process and does not always progress smoothly. Some individuals resort to intensified magical thinking and blame others for their predicament in a strange mixture of paranoid ideas and grandiose distortions. Occasionally patients retire to a state of permanent dependency, becoming passive-aggressive in their interactions with caregivers and significant others. For some, depression deepens, making death by suicide a real possibility. Reason and simple encouragement are only of limited assistance in dealing with the patient's rage at the world, a pervasive sense of worthlessness, and utter despair. However, in most patients there are islands of hope and personality organization still intact. These provide the basis for patients' use of the skills and activities they still have. Renewed assertive activity serves to preserve self-esteem and provides a bridge to the world of active rehabilitation.

## Coping, Stabilization, Struggle for New Self

The coping and stabilization stage emerges quietly from the preceding crisis. As the struggle continues, patients gradually extend their repertoire of limited activities, gaining gratification through ability to meet some self-care needs. Self-esteem is slowly restored through activity and skill acquisition. Rosalind Chambers (1966), stricken with polio and confined for months to an iron lung, writes of this stage:

> It seems essential to a man's self-respect that he should find himself of use, and it is no less necessary for a woman. On becoming disabled the man or woman has probably lost the power to continue his/her previous job, and a wife the power to look after her family. Both are traumatic experiences, and *something else must be found as soon as possible* [emphasis added]. Anything will do at first. Obviously the degree of paralysis affects the ease with which suitable tasks can be found, but there is always *something*. I used to encourage people to discuss their plans for the future with me, and it seemed to help them sort out their ideas. Later, when the victim improves his condition, it is time to look around *for more things to do* (emphasis added). (pp. 25–26)

This phase thus begins a pilgrimage to find a new self. Rehabilitation, a kind of relearning of new tasks and functions, becomes the central life effort. The individual regains increasing interest in and capacity to think about the world outside his or her immediate needs. At times this "rediscovery" of the world can be quite touching, as Ms. Chambers describes:

> From the months in the general hospital my most vivid recollection is of the first time I was taken out of the ward and downstairs to the nurses' hostel to have a cup of coffee. On the way down a door was open to the garden and I saw the grass. We stopped, and I stared in astonishment and exaltation. Its greenness was of a quality beyond memory and beyond imagination. I drank it in, and it was as though my body had lacked some mysterious chlorophyll of its own which it now recognized and absorbed. That moment should be put on the scales against all the previous pain and frustration and humiliation; and I think the scales would balance. (p. 27)

As the individual becomes more involved with rehabilitative activities and relationships, the regressive tendencies subside. Yet, with each new problem and each new demand encountered, patients are confronted with new vulnerabilities and sensitivities. That others enjoy the intactness of their bodies while the physically impaired person struggles to master every new task can elicit in the latter periodic flashes of anger. The "touchiness" often noted in individuals with major physical impairments results from this struggle, amplified by the fear that others will not recognize that their value as unique individuals and their potential to be living partners or productive workers are intact. These issues remain for the lifetime of the physically impaired person.

# Contingencies

The details of the course and outcome of the long journey of rehabilitation for a particular individual will be influenced by that person's past life experience and his or her repertoire of strengths and weaknesses. Current social, familial, contextual, and cultural relationships will also alter the intensity of response. Although these factors are not the focus of the book, they cannot be ignored. Details of how varied the individual reactions may be to a specific impairment, such as paraplegia, may be found in the rehabilitation literature (Bracken and Bernstein 1980). Because the hands, face, and genitalia hold special meaning to a person's identity and sense of personal attractiveness, impairments of these body parts will have added psychological impact (Castelnuovo-Tedesco 1984). Factors to be considered also include the natural history of the underlying disease or trauma, and whether it is congenital or acquired. Some impairments are ominously progressive, and some unpredictably progressive, while others are stationary or improve over time.

The meaning of a specific impairment to an individual also varies widely. An acquired blindness has a different meaning for a painter than for a poet. An acquired spinal cord injury is experienced differently by a basketball star than a law student. The age of the patient is also an important variable. Families will also respond differentially to different injuries. No single factor determines which individuals will rise to the challenge of their rehabilitation with dramatically vigorous and competent responses and which might be permanently shattered by the impairment, withdraw from the world, and give up apathetically, or die in the face of a debilitating depression.

Regardless of this multiplicity of factors, each individual in rehabilitation is faced with the overwhelming task of confronting loss and finding new solutions to the problems of functional limitations. Each individual must build a new identity and a new way of dealing with the world. The process of working through these issues cannot be rushed but must occur in an individualized mix of stimulus and reward, small success and failure.

Hamburg and Adams (1967) have focused on coping behavior: that is, "[the individual in rehabilitation] keeping distress within manageable limits; maintaining a sense of personal worth; restoring relations with significant other people; enhancing prospects for recovery of bodily functions; and increasing the likelihood of working out a personally valued and socially acceptable situation long after maximum physical recovery has been attained" (p. 278). This one-step-at-a-time process may be a matter of weeks, months, or years, depending on the patient and the problems. The context that facilitates this rehabilitative process and the people that create that context are the subject of the remainder of this book.

## After Being Paralyzed From the Neck Down for Twenty Years, Mr. Wallace Gets a Chin-Operated Motorized Wheelchair

For the first time in twenty years
he is mobile, roaring through corridors,
bouncing off walls, out of control,
breaking doorways, tables, chairs,
and regulations. The hallways stretch out
behind him, startled, amazed,
their plaster and wallpaper gaping,
while somewhere far off,
arms spastically flailing,
the small nurses continue to call:
*Mr. Wallace . . . Mr. Wallace . . .*

Eventually he'll listen to reason
and go quietly back to his room,
docile, repentant, and sheepish, promising
not to disappoint them again.
The day shift will sigh and go home.
But, in the evening, between feeding and bedtime,
when they've finally left him alone,
he'll roar over to the corner
and crash through the window
stopping only to watch
the last geese rising,
rising by the light of the snow.

*Ronald Wallace*

# 4

# Developmental Considerations

## A Developmental Point of View

In reviewing the variety of settings and situations in which caregiving occurs, it is apparent that many aspects of the transactions between caregivers and a patient with a catastrophic injury are "developmental" in the broadest sense; that is, they resemble in form and dynamic the interactions between a parent and a child. The critical distinction here, of course, is that the patient generally is usually not a child but a physically impaired adult struggling to regain lost adult functions and status. Developmental models have great power and also strict limitations. As in psychotherapy, there is no demeaning of adults by likening affects or dynamics to those of children. A second caveat is that developmental models are constructed from and thus normalized only for the unimpaired, as Gliedman and Roth (1980) have emphasized. Nevertheless, certain aspects and qualities of the "caregiving encounter" so reliably echo themes best seen within a developmental framework that use of the model seems justified.

As relationships between parent and child evolve over time (especially as regards decision making and autonomy), so do relationships between physically impaired adults and their caregivers during rehabilitation processes. In this chapter we explore these parallels as a guide to better understanding of caregiver reactions. The alert reader will discover in these encounters the biases of the committee's value system. Any transaction between patient and caregiver will contain a value-laden message that communicates to the patient what kind of a place the facility is and how in turn the patient is seen and understood by staff members and the facility as a whole. Caregivers become the important bearers of an implied value system in any facility or institution in which they work. Such a transmission of values can be clearly perceived using a developmental model.

## Caring for the Immobilized Patient

Consider this personal statement of a quadriplegic young man describing the early aftermath of his cervical cord injury:

> The fourth experience that I can link to adjustment was the helpless feeling. In most cases of cervical injury, there is a total paralysis for many weeks, depending on how high the lesion and how extensive the damage. During those weeks of total paralysis, you can do nothing for yourself. For me, those first weeks were spent lying in traction on a Stryker frame staring at the ceiling for four hours, then at the floor for four hours, turned every four hours night and day. Someone had to feed me, bathe me, brush my teeth, help my bowels move, even scratch my nose. I was totally dependent on other people to do everything for me. It is hard to move from complete dependence to complete reliance. However, it is an adjustment you must make or frustration will eat at you until anger at the whole world turns to depression. You can develop an "I don't care" attitude or even a "death wish." When a person gives up at this point, his road to recovery will be that much longer and harder. *This is why I emphasize the importance of hope. Nothing or no one should be allowed to take it away or destroy it* . . . [emphasis added]. At this point an injured person is so disoriented and confused that hope and faith or denial is one of the most important psychological attitudes he or she can have. (Caywood 1974, p. 22)

The total (regressive) physical dependency of such a patient on his caregivers is not only factual but sobering as well. In this situation, one's bodily needs have been reduced to a stage of infantilized dependency in which all physical needs are met from the outside. Such a situation puts the caregiver in a jarring paradox, for one must handle the body of a patient as if the patient were an infant while responding to the person in the broad sense as an adult. The dangers of infantilizing bodily care, and inadvertently the person, are ubiquitous. Although medical care through this period must have a nurturing quality, it must also avoid being condescending or belittling to the patient, who submits to its inevitable indignities with adult sensibilities and experiential memory intact. What sustains the patient through such a time of forced immobilization? Denial certainly, but a sense of hope as well that serves as a critical motivation throughout this initial period. (Later, these initial hopes are reshaped by the reality of the situation.)

The above-mentioned patient underscores a caregiving attitude that closely parallels the child/mother transactions of infancy:

> Hope is both the earliest and most indispensable virtue inherent in the state of being alive . . . if life is to be sustained hope must remain, even when confidence is wounded, trust impaired. . . . In infancy, hope relies for its beginnings on the new being's first encounter with trustworthy persons. (Erikson 1964, p. 115)

A dependency-producing, catastrophic physical impairment turns back a developmental clock to a stage thus paralleling early childhood experiences of trustworthiness. Caregivers are now called upon to sustain hope and to assist the patient in believing that the future can be better than the present. Each patient needs to believe (as did each of us as small children) that we all are, or can become, more than we seem to be at present. Thus, the good caregiver in such situations conveys a spirit of balanced, realistic optimism and brings to the bedside an attitude that things can change.

Such a goal sounds laudable indeed, but determining how to replicate the essential features of such balanced nurturance is far from easy. Daily working rituals provide subtle and ubiquitous reminders of inequalities and losses. Consider as simple an exchange as eye contact. Certainly no one wishes to be "looked down upon," and yet the world of wheelchair vision functions at least a foot lower than the majority of visual transactions. Whenever possible, the sensitive caregiver takes a position at eye level with the patient to avoid the subtle condescending message and to allow ease in exchange. This "little grace" requires repetitive time and effort. Similarly, persons in wheelchairs are best approached from the front prefaced by identification and introduction, rather than suddenly set in motion from behind with neither elegance nor warning. Simple graces of social exchange require adjustments when the eye level, mobility, or perception is so altered that more traditional exchanges acquire implications of condescension, inequality, or paternalism. The message to be conveyed is equality in humanity, if not identity in role or functional ability.

Nevertheless, the caregiver has an intact body and the patient an impaired one, and thus the patient is inevitably "one down" in many transactions. What else can the caregiver do to avoid unnecessary and unintentional bias? Physician-poet William Carlos Williams provides an additional touch point: "An important part of a physician's [caregiver's] life is spent listening to people tell you their stories; and in return, they want to hear your story of what their story means" (Coles 1989, p. 105). Williams reminds us that every patient has a "life story" (by definition the essence of development) as well as an impairment. In the mutual sharing of life experience, both patient and caregiver can find some common human ground, and thus a fraternal equality of sorts gives the caregiving task an added dimension of dignity. No longer is the patient just defined by the anatomic lesion ("the quadriplegic") but by a life story, a common human past. We do not here suggest a trite, nonprofessional familiarity between a physically impaired person and his or her caregivers; nor are we trying to make all caregivers into amateur psychotherapists. Only bear in mind that each patient brings all of his or her former life experiences into this present struggle, and these stories, the telling and the listening, bring an otherwise awkward relationship closer into balance, offsetting much of the painful regression and dependency of the initial caregiving needs and affront to adult autonomy. Dr. Williams again:

> But most of my patients . . . they want to gab away, but they're not sure how to get going. They're in trouble and that is when you're eager to look into things deep, real deep. I wouldn't walk away from those kinds of talks for anything; I come away from them so damn stirred myself. . . . You get stopped in your tracks by something the patient says, and it takes time to let its way through your head and heart. (Coles 1989, p. 104)

Another tactic that parallels a parent/child interaction in the daily care of the immobilized patient is the introduction of novelty. Immobilization can lead at times to a kind of sensory deprivation. Things can become too routine, dull, and thus boring. The astute caregiver, much like the alert parent, looks for ways to introduce novelty into these routines. In addition to the notion of newness, every parent intuitively realizes that there are certain "golden moments" with their offspring when a word or a gesture has a crucial influence. Thus does an ordinary interaction achieve extraordinary impact. Consider the following example of doing the "right thing at the right time":

> Michael Naranjo . . . was blinded by a grenade in the Vietnam war. Mr. Naranjo has become an accomplished sculptor despite his loss of eyesight. Interested in sculpture from childhood, he described in an interview the initial moment of his recovery through applying himself again to his interest. He had spent about three or four weeks in a hospital bed in Japan: ". . . I was very tired of just lying there. I couldn't get out of bed because my right arm was tied down. I asked for some modelling clay. Water based clay. While I was lying there in bed, I made a little worm, a goldfish, and then I made a stick figure of 'The Thinker.' Then I made a squirrel with a nut in his hand. In Fitzimmons General Hospital in Denver, I asked for some oil-based clay. I made this Indian

whipping a horse across a plain. His braids are flying behind him, and so are the tail and mane of his horse. Once I made that Indian and horse, I truly knew that I could sculpt again." (Smith and Plimpton 1989, p. 46)

Simple, earthy clay (introduced at the right time) gave the patient the impetus to again pursue his life's ambition. A more apt metaphor of ascendancy from the concrete to the transcendent could hardly be conceived.

Along similar developmental lines, children confined to intensive care units need not only the novelty of new sensory input but also the familiarity of records, stories, and daily rituals to help provide crucial links of continuity with their past. The astute caregiver uses the patient and the family as one's resource for this information and as an ally in arranging periodic treats and surprises to break up the relentless inpatient routines.

## Movement From Dependency
## Toward Autonomy

As rehabilitation proceeds, patients are frequently relearning to use functions in one or more limbs. This includes patients in wheelchairs but also patients with braces and a variety of prosthetic aids. A parallel exists here with development, as the child learns (for the first time) to walk and master increasingly difficult motor tasks with hands and feet. There is always a succession of successes and failures as the patient works with his or her physical and occupational therapists to achieve maximal functioning. The drive to remaster these skills parallels the child's will to master the immediate environment, however simple or technical. The "good" caregiver, like the good parent, encourages this inner drive for mastery by allowing and rewarding as much autonomy as is useful and practical at a particular stage. No caregiver need solve a problem or do something for a patient that that person can do for himself or herself. Even in small things, recovering patients can be given as many choices as they can handle. The optimal milieu is arranged so that problem solving is developmentally appropriate, mutually facilitated, and firmly reinforced and rewarded.

Any caregiving environment is optimally flexible if there is always something left to do or to change. The best rehabilitation programs give one a sense of ragged edges and unfinished business that may not always be visually satisfying but that seem vital to the success of patient progress overall. Nancy Kerr is a psychologist with an acquired disability who addresses this phase of her own experience:

> I had a physical therapist who, while working within the framework of the medical prescription, let me make every decision possible concerning therapy. To be sure, the initial options were small, like which exercises we'd work on first, or which chair I'd learn to transfer into next. Later, I was encouraged to make more crucial decisions such as whether it was more important to me—with my plans and obligations—to be a resident patient or a day patient. (Kerr 1977, p. 51)

Physically impaired patients, in recapturing their own earlier sense of autonomy and will, may not initially do so very gracefully. A sense of bitterness and negativism often accompanies their first efforts. The skillful caregiver recognizes that a person's feelings do not come in pleasant and tidy packages. The caregiver accepts the bitterness as not personal while continuing to foster the patient's more healthy drive toward continued improvement. In other words, the caregiver "hears" the message of determination and may choose to accept the static of bitterness as a normal, indeed necessary, component. By selectively focusing on the positive, the caregiver sustains the patient's "new" (i.e., reemergent adult) drive to reestablish ever more control over his or her life.

The developmental task for caregiver, as for parent, is to foster autonomy and competence by setting realistic, incremental goals along the way and assuaging temporary defeats in a supportive manner. In practical terms this means patients are never intentionally or unnecessarily diminished by anything we say or do. This approach also suggests that caregivers explain honestly and frequently *what* they are doing and *why* they are doing it.

> Perhaps the most common way of telling the patient that he is a machine in the shop for repair is the habit some staffers have of communicating with the attendant pushing the wheelchair instead of with the patient himself. The patient thus finds himself sandwiched between two white coats with one asking the other, "Now where does she go?" (Kerr 1977, p. 53)

Such an attitude means we should not be blandly reassuring or subtly condescending, for both attitudes have in common a diminishment of the patient. It implies that caregivers maintain realistic expectations and are not easily defeated by the inevitable failures along the way. All these admonitions sound much like Winnicott's "good-enough mothering" of developmental theory—that is, a persistence of timing and skill sufficient for the task at hand. Skilled caregivers of all disciplines are found to possess these critical perceptive, limiting, and supportive qualities.

## Movement From Hospital to Community

Even as we all at one time left home in various stages of development, first to attend school and later to become financially independent, so too does the patient in rehabilitation make this crucial developmental step at some time, possibly in stages. Moving along the rehabilitation pathway means moving to a more pressured, high-expectation environment and eventually confronting the relative harshness of the nondisabled world. Paralleling the adolescent's "identity crisis" in confronting the awesome tasks of mastering job and school, as well as sexual feelings, without parental protection, so too patients leaving rehabilitation settings face major issues in these areas when they leave the shelter of the institution.

In our society of exaggerated independence, any person needing continual assistance is likely to encounter problems of status, moral worth, and precarious identity (Thomas 1982). The dangers of this transition to the community for such a person are relative exclusion from the mainstream, constriction of social role, and limitation of opportunity. Turner and Beiser (1990) have recently shown in a large community sample that physically disabled people show much higher rates of both depressive symptoms and major depressive disorder than do their nondisabled counterparts. One of the major difficulties for many people who have suffered disabling conditions is the task of regaining a sense of purpose. Keith (1988) documents that some rehabilitation settings do not provide many opportunities for adequate independent behavior prior to discharge. The transition to "normal" life may be formidable indeed. Cogswell (1968) has noted that the interval required to return to work posthospital was in the range of one to several years, although most of the individuals in her sample eventually did return to gainful employment:

> It is easier to establish and maintain a positive self-image in the sheltered social environment of the hospital than in the world outside. When paraplegics return to their homes and communities, definitions of their disability as a social stigma reach the height of salience. This common problem apparently orders their course of socialization. (p. 12)

It takes time for individuals with a physical disability to reorder their future life in accordance with their new limitations. Such a transition is analogous to what Erikson (1975) has called the "psychosocial moratorium of adolescence." Every young person needs time to determine in what direction to go. This is also true for the individual with a life-altering physical impairment. A 55-year-old psychologist, Dr. K., was rendered quadriplegic as the result of a swimming accident in his youth. After his immediate recovery, he reached a plateau in his rehabilitation and recalls this phase as follows:

> I had reached a point in my life for several years where I badly needed and wanted to get free from being housebound to being a productive citizen. I was reasonably bright, but I was lost as to how to go about getting for myself the help I needed. In essence, I got lost in the social network cracks and was buried there for a long period of time. The help eventually came because a public health nurse recognized my potential and my need to get out and do something. She urged me to go back to school. She also facilitated this process by helping me connect with the right resource. I then eventually got into graduate school and got my Ph.D. in psychology. (personal communication)

Dr. K's story implies a kind of moratorium in moving from the confines of his home back out into the world. This can be a lonely time as the individual mobilizes his or her resources to face this task. Of course the role of the caregiver is crucial in knowing when to begin to encourage such a move. Caregivers will recognize the time it takes to make this transition. They should try not to expect too much too soon, nor allow former patients to languish in an isolated, passive community existence. Like good parents, caregivers help such individuals see that they can do more and be more than they are at present. A sense of the future is always part of any moment-to-moment interaction with a physically impaired person returning to the community (just as it is with an adolescent). At the same time, and again paralleling a parental role, caregivers assist the individual with an impairment to anticipate the uncertainty of this struggle. Thus they provide for the continuity of care so that the former patient has a safe place to periodically retreat to for "emotional refuelling" (to borrow a term of Margaret Mahler's). For at times individuals with a physical impairment need to be allowed to move backward temporarily while they are, on the whole, moving forward. As in the development of most adolescents, one's course is marked by uneven movement, characterized by some success, some failure, and occasionally plateaus of relative stability. The process is rarely smooth or neatly completed. It is often punctuated (as in the teenage years) by crises, regression, and occasional breakthroughs.

## Human Values and the Developmental View

The developmental parallels between the care of a recovering person with a severe physical impairment and the care good parents give to their own children have been drawn in this chapter. We conclude with some brief comments about the value system upon which such a developmental viewpoint rests.

Perhaps the reader has already detected the value system implicit in this schema. In their transactions with patients, caregivers strive to convey a sense of hope, a respect for the individuality and autonomy of each person, a wish to motivate new purpose and aims for each individual, and the recognition that continuity of care and extracurricular social support networks in the community are vital to any rehabilitation effort. Caregivers learn to tolerate failure both in themselves and in their patients while maintaining their professional relationship of support and encouragement. All such activities sound like, again, not only good clinical care but good parenting as well. Developmental models allow explanations of processes (and also moods, personality conflicts, and peculiar psychological gaps) that ease the path for patient and provider alike, and soften the bumps with anticipation and prospective planning.

Erikson pointed out that the provision of care itself is an essential developmental stage in the drama of the human life cycle. In the transactions that occur between caregiver and physically impaired person, each participates in this drama in a fundamentally human fashion. Erikson (1964) described the adult man or woman as "so constituted as to need to be needed lest he or she suffer the mental deformation of self-absorption, in which man becomes his own infant or pet" (p. 130). Caring for impaired individuals is one of many ways that such a stage in human development can come to fruition. For all of us, as caregivers, "the challenge emanates from what we have generated and from what now must be brought up, guarded, preserved, and eventually transcended" (Erikson 1964, p. 131).

# SECTION 2:
# CLINICAL APPLICATIONS

### From My Mouth to God's Ear

"How do you do it?" they ask
"I could never stand it!"
"It must be so depressing."

I smile modestly, shrug off their comments.
How can I speak of these aching times?
The moments when it seems
      that everyone is dying
And I must somehow gather the strength to go to
them,
      attend to them,
      get inside their feelings enough
  to say the right thing.
I am haunted by memories of children I have
watched
      turning blue from the feet up.

As I listen to their slow, irregular gasps
      I pray that their pain
      is not so great as that of those
      who listen, and watch.
From parents I hear the anguished cry:
      Why me?
      How could this happen to my child?

Helpless to explain, I am certain only of this:
There is nothing anyone could possibly do which
could be deserving of this.

*Margaret Stuber, M.D.*

# 5

# Caregiver Reactions

"How do you do it? I could never stand that kind of work!" Most caregivers have heard such comments. Whether they reflect awe and respect, or amazed disbelief, these responses of others to rehabilitation work should properly mark caregivers as a special and heroic group of people who have undertaken an enormous, and occasionally misunderstood, task. Most caregivers do not *feel* particularly heroic, but they *do feel* things intensely as they involve themselves with physically impaired persons and their families. Over time, caregivers learn to value the deep satisfactions that come with this kind of human involvement, as well as tolerate the disappointments and frustrations that inevitably accompany this endeavor.

In this chapter we have two main goals. The first is to expand and illustrate several of the psychological concepts mentioned earlier in this monograph. The reactions of caregivers arise within a complex array of multidimensional, transactional relationships. Specific psychodynamic concepts that pertain to caregivers (such as regression, splitting, and "selfobject") will be illustrated as well. A better understanding of these concepts can broaden caregivers' understanding and make their work more empathic and meaningful.

Our second goal in this chapter is to describe more specifically some common reactions of caregivers and consultants working with individuals with physical impairments and their families. These will be presented in a somewhat artificial manner for the sake of clarity. Human experience is complicated, multifaceted, and, above all, holistic, whether we are discussing our reactions to people with body-altering impairments or to anyone else. Reactions do not occur in neat categorical entities. For instance, if one is irritated at a patient or family member, one usually feels some guilt as well for having this negative reaction.

Reactions to patients (and their reactions to us) come and go, build and recede, and can be hidden from awareness. In this chapter we will essentially provide "snapshots" of what in reality is a moving picture.

## Psychological/Psychodynamic Concepts

### Introspection, Empathy, and the Transactional Process

Every caregiver in any setting is carrying on relationships not only with patients and their families but with a variety of professional colleagues, some of whom are peers, and others of whom are in positions of authority. Thus, caregiver reactions are going to be a constant panoply of response to multiple situations and stimuli. In addition, each of us brings to our caregiving tasks particular background experiences and personality styles. Caregivers react to patients in terms of the meaning of that behavior (meanings of which one is not always conscious). Less commonly known, however, is that patients (with or without impairments) generate in professional and family caregivers emotional reactions that are similar to the patients' own inner emotional states. If attention is paid to the kinds of feelings patients elicit in us, we gain valuable clues to our patients' emotional situation. This is not always simple. Nevertheless, paying attention to this dimension of our work gives us an additional tool with which to assist our patients.

This "listening to our own signals" (termed *introspection*) is one of the major ways learning about the inner emotional state of another person occurs. There are obvious hazards and obstacles. First, caregivers may be too busy to engage in this kind of reflective activity; the moment-to-moment demands of work may be too great. Second, caregivers may resist recognizing some negative feelings about their patients, feeling that these are inappropriate. We may instinctively feel guilty for having some of the feelings because they do not square with a concept of ourselves as competent caregivers. Third, caregivers' feelings about a patient may not be accurate. Instead, they may be coming from some other relationships, displaced onto this interaction.

How can a caregiver know whether the responses a patient is eliciting are a clue to that person's emotional state? Practice in the art of listening to oneself helps, but for most, the solution to each of these three obstacles can be the same: the *team meeting*. The team meeting should serve as a mechanism to support our honest efforts to get in touch with our own feelings about a particular patient. It allows time for us to check out perceptions with others on the team. "Is this the way patient X makes you feel too?" The caregiver is given permission to share some less savory reactions in a safe atmosphere where he or she can verbalize reactions instead of letting them simmer. Team meetings do not serve as group therapy for the caregivers; rather they provide sophisticated peer supervision and group learning. The focus is always on the patient, and caregiver responses to the patient are examined in the service of patient care, not caregiver therapy, as in the following example:

> A 22-year-old woman was several weeks into her rehabilitation for a severe injury that rendered her right leg nonfunctional. She showed a persistent wish to be cooperative with her caregivers, never complaining, and always presented them with a cheerful smile. Yet there was something in her demeanor that left her caregivers unsettled and unhappy. At a team meeting, one of the staff mentioned that the patient's smile seemed brave but "fake," and she found herself, as a caregiver, irritated by the patient's artificial cheerfulness and attempts to act as if nothing very serious was wrong. Other caregivers concurred, stating they often felt exhausted after caring for her. Further team discussion led to the notion that this woman might be rather depressed underneath her "brave front" and that the team needed to keep this issue in mind as they cared for her. Several days later, one of the patient's caregivers noted that this woman was getting irritated that her leg brace wouldn't lock into place correctly. The caregiver said lightly, "Whew, I'm glad to see you can get angry once in a while. I was wondering where all those feelings were." The patient looked startled, then broke down in tears as she confessed how much she hated the whole lousy business of being in the hospital.

Every hospital contains a certain number of "smiling" depressed patients. The best way to detect them is to catch a sense of one's own reactions in interacting with these patients. A let down in mood or slight irritability in the interaction can often be the first clue to the inner experience of the patient.

Similarly, there are times in care settings when a caregiver's sense of "confusion" in listening to the patient will be the first tip-off that this patient is moving into a delirious state. Patients with severe injuries are prone to acute delirious states in the early stages of their care. The astute caregiver may first notice only that what the patient is saying does not quite make sense. Being confused is an important diagnostic clue in the caregiver to the patient's mental status. However, caution is advised in verbalizing caregiver reactions or making interpretations of the patient's feelings directly back to the patient. Patients are often not consciously aware of the feelings and may become enraged at being presented with interpretations they have not requested. It is best to check out reactions with other caregivers at the team meeting and use this feedback in developing a consistent care plan that takes the reactions into account. Often the assistance of a consultant is useful when particular patients or their families arouse intense feelings in a number of the caregiving staff.

## Regression and Splitting

Transactions over time between a patient with a physical impairment and a variety of caregivers can become complicated. A particularly difficult interaction is one in which patients relate to caregivers as though some were "good" and others "bad," creating divisions in the team. This is usually called *splitting*. A patient may thus tend to "scapegoat" certain caregivers while lavishing praise on others. Such splits can be powerful enough to cause staff to take sides, creating tension and competition in the team. Families may also be divided, competing with staff and relatives to be the "good" caregiver. Again, the team meeting is the optimal place to recognize and deal with this pattern. The reasons patients tend to do this are myriad and are often unrecognized by the patients. The experienced caregiver learns not to take too seriously either criticism or praise from any given patient and is ready to be the recipient of a variety of feelings from the physically impaired patient that often erupt unexpectedly and without explanation. Caregivers learn to operate emotionally in a kind of semidarkness, with faith that momentary upsets will be worked through over time.

The protective regression common to humans faced by an enormous threat contributes to the phenomena of splitting. Regression allows one to return, in behavior and attitudes, to an earlier time in development, when life was simpler and more secure, and parents were available to share in one's troubles. All seriously ill people become regressed, self-oriented, occasionally demanding, and at times impulsive. In such a state, the ability to hold mixed, or ambivalent, feelings seems too complicated and demanding. Indeed, recent child development research shows that normal children cannot report mixed feelings about another person until they are about 10 years old (Harter and Buddin 1987). Relationships can therefore be easily divided into polarized categories (i.e., all good or all bad).

Reality issues can also contribute to splitting, such as when caregivers must carry out tasks that are medically important but elicit pain and distress in the patient (e.g., painful dressing changes in a burned patient). Staff need to support each other and rotate roles so that particular staff are not seen as cruel "ogres" by the patient.

## Boundaries (Aladdin's Perfect Genie)

Occasionally caregivers are pleasantly surprised by the intensity of faith that patients or family members have in caregivers' ability to ease pain, cure disease, or reverse the steady deterioration of aging. Yet such admiration generally comes at a high price: caregivers must be perfect and always make themselves available to the patient, providing instant service and marvelous solutions. Anything short of this is not enough. Caregivers may come to feel like genies—capable of any magic, but slaves to the patient's slightest whim. Another manifestation of this same phenomenon is the experience of having patients demand endless enthusiastic applause for their latest small accomplishment. These are variants of the boundary issues referred to in Chapter 2. This type of relationship is rather common between severely physically impaired patients and their caregivers during the early part of rehabilitation. Patients behave as if patient and caregiver are psychologically one, with the caregiver acknowledged to exist only as an extension of the patient, without a separate mind or will. This attitude can be confusing and maddening to the caregiver, contributing to a sense of burnout, because it is impossible truly to please such a patient. Such interactions are common, however, as they allow the seriously threatened patient to regain a sense of power and capability to influence the world, indirectly leading to a restoration of self-esteem damaged by the impairment.

Even an experienced consultant may have problems with patients who have this type of expectation, as in the following case:

> A 35-year-old woman whose right arm was severely injured in a car accident was initially grateful for the opportunity to discuss her situation with a psychiatric consultant. This was heartening to the consultant, but it seemed a bit excessive. Nevertheless, the woman seemed to use the counseling well and dealt realistically with the various issues she faced as her rehabilitation proceeded. After 8 to 10 sessions, her attitude toward the consultant turned abruptly hostile and she became as negative as she had formerly been positive. The consultant was baffled by this sudden change and by his inability to anticipate it. He speculated that this patient's gratitude to him assumed he would restore some aspect of her disabled right arm (a kind of bargaining). But she refused to talk further, leaving him unable to work this through or help this patient understand herself better.

This vignette also illustrates the fact that failure is a reality for all who do this work.

# Specific Caregiver Reactions

In the second portion of this chapter we present in a dialectic style some common responses of caregivers in transaction with people who have physical impairments. Reactions are described along a continuum, the extremes of which are usually undesirable. The caregiver's challenge is to find the balance or desirable middle ground between the extremes. Although focusing specifically on professional caregivers and their patients, these reactions are also usually operative in interactions between staff and family, and between patients and their families.

## Optimal Staff Involvement: Distance Versus Identification

A common point of discussion among caregivers is the amount of professional distance that is appropriate in working with people with physical impairments. Getting too close means losing perspective and leverage, while too much distance makes one emotionally unavailable. A major determinant of the distance taken is caregiver anxiety.

Anxiety is an expectable response to work with people with physical impairments. A major source of anxiety for caregivers is the sense of vulnerability experienced by all individuals when confronted by the reality of an impairment. The person with a physical impairment is generally experienced as a threat to one's own body integrity. Most individuals respond to such a threat with anxiety, which may manifest as a feeling of vague uneasiness, a desire to escape, or an almost superstitious fear of contagion. These reactions are significantly stronger if the patient resembles the caregiver in pertinent ways, such as age, background, race, or education. Such similarities facilitate *identification*, a sense that "this might be me." A certain level of selective identification is necessary for a true empathic understanding. However, over-identification can create such an overwhelming sense of threat that the caregiver withdraws, shutting off the possibility of empathy.

A common distancing response to this sense of vulnerability is to define the patient as significantly different from the caregiver. Psychological withdrawal is often accompanied by physical avoidance; both reactions serve to put distance between one's self and the threat. Intellectual mastery of a specific area can provide a sense of competence and thus control anxiety. However, this kind of mastery can lead to such a rigid division between the caregiver and the patient that no empathy is possible. Patients begin to be labeled by their impairment, such as "the double amputee in the corner room." However, optimal distance is necessary to maintain a perspective on the entire process of the work. Caregivers cannot be effective when they are emotionally isolated in the service of managing anxiety *or* overinvolved in the care of patients, and thus losing sight of the long-range goals of treatment.

Another form of distancing is manifested at an institutional level by uniforms, use of titles, and other more subtle forms of differentiation. Some role definition is essential in establishing work relationships, just as psychological distancing is necessary to avoid overidentification. However, distancing requires balance lest caregivers' role identities interfere with their ability to work together with a professional perspective.

The balance between isolating distance and overinvolvement is demonstrated in the rehabilitation of a young child in the following example:

> A 5-year-old child was hospitalized for severe burns with accompanying facial disfigurement. The child's chronic pain and irritability seemed to push the caregivers away from genuine involvement with her as a person. The parents noted the impersonal nature of the care she was receiving and in some alarm complained to the head nurse. The bedside caregivers in turn complained that the child was so negative and irritable that appropriate responses were nearly impossible. After some reflection on this issue at a team meeting, the head nurse suggested that the parents bring pictures of the child before the fire. The parents also taught the caregivers about their child's interests through drawings and taped music. Gradually, this child became a person, rather than a disagreeable "case." The staff began to work with her more comfortably, and the child in turn became more responsive to her caregivers.

## Sexual Issues in Persons With Physical Impairments

Sexuality is a core human experience. Sexual activity constitutes a crucial way one confirms one's self-esteem as a worthy adult and one's capability for giving as well as receiving pleasure and affection. For the physically impaired person, sexual activity may constitute an even more vital source of self-affirmation than before the injury. Yet anxieties about one's ability and capacity to perform sexually are often pronounced and thus greatly affect one's overall sense of self-worth.

A brief examination of studies of male patients with spinal cord injuries shows that over 75% of these patients retain erectile capacity. Preservation of the capacity for ejaculation is less clear. Spinal cord–injured women usually resume their menses within 6 months. Fertility remains unimpaired, so contraception is a subject that must be addressed. While in all spinal cord–injured individuals sexual sensation is greatly diminished, some degree of autonomically monitored activity seems to provide an awareness of erection and orgasm (Smith 1981).

Sexual feelings and concerns in the patient with a physical impairment constitute a particularly troublesome area for the patient's caregiver, because as care providers we can easily retreat to a position of seeing the person in our charge as "asexual," thus negating or minimizing this patient's future potential for intimate relationships. Caregivers are often unaware of this reaction, which appears to spring from the deeply rooted aversion to visible disability discussed earlier (see Chapter 2). Certain situations, such as those involving patients with head injuries who are disinhibited or young men with spinal cord injuries, can be particularly difficult for caregivers. Safilios-Rothchild (1970) suggested that "the main type of aversion (to disabled persons) is 'aesthetic-sexual,'" concluding that "while the non-disabled tend to be cooperative and understanding when it comes to the occupational world, they close their ears to the disabled's attempts to gain social acceptance and marriage eligibility" (p. 128). Despite a truly empathic relationship in other areas, for many "the mere thought of an intimate relationship with a disabled person may be an offensive idea which conjures up feelings of disgust or repugnance" (Hahn 1981, p. 224). These responses interfere with empathy for the patient, distancing the caregiver. They may also interfere with complete patient rehabilitation if they create a blind spot for the sexual teaching that is indicated for most neurological or musculoskeletal impairments. Caregivers who are disturbed by the idea of sexual activity in a patient with a physical impairment are less likely to be capable of a neutral advocacy role in this important area of function.

Many patient-caregiver encounters are male-female. Moreover, the caregiving transactions are bodily transactions that put both participants into close physical contact. Over time these bodily ministrations can take on sexual overtones, putting both caregiver and patient under new instinctual pressure. This in turn can influence the total relationship, adding stress to what the caregiver feels and anxiety to what the patient feels.

The following vignette illustrates how both the loss of bodily function and the loss of an important relationship can get channeled into a sexualized behavior that becomes disruptive to care:

A 25-year-old male patient with multiple injuries resulting from a severe car accident is confined to a body cast and has been in the hospital for 2 months. The staff know his wife has recently separated from him. They also note that he begins taking "liberties" in his interactions during bathing and routine care (i.e., by slapping nurses on the buttocks as they walk past his bed).

It would be difficult for any caregiver faced with this behavior to empathically see beyond it. Some reflective discussion at a team meeting, perhaps with the assistance of a mental health consultant, would allow caregivers to work out a consistent response plan that can bring resolution to this situation for the caregiver and help to the patient.

Some caregivers, however, will find that their discomfort with a patient's sexuality has to do with their attraction to individual patients. Given the intimacy and length of interactions between patients and caregivers, it is not surprising that such strong feelings develop. Unfortunately, these responses often take on a paternalistic character. Caregivers feeling noble and generous may wish to rescue the patients. Some caregivers may also see this as an opportunity to enter a relationship that allows them a great deal of control or power. These are dangerous reasons to enter any relationship and are unethical in some situations. Although team meetings may seem an odd place to discuss such feelings, they provide a useful forum for helping caregivers recognize the reasons for these responses. A discussion may aid in thinking about, rather than acting on, such impulses (DeLoach and Green 1981). Psychiatric consultation to the team or caregiver can also be useful in such circumstances.

## Responsibility and Powerlessness: Whose Life Is It, Anyway?

Another source of anxiety for caregivers is their sense of responsibility for the people who depend upon them. Caregivers vary in their experience of responsibility and power in regard to individuals with physical impairment. Some may feel that the total outcome of the person's care is their responsibility and is dependent solely upon their efforts and skill. Although this is empowering to the caregiver, it is ultimately destructive to the autonomy of the physically impaired person. It thus undermines the purpose of the work. A caregiver can take pleasure in the accomplishments of the disabled person, and share in a sense of power, without taking control.

An inflated sense of responsibility can also present difficulties if the caregiver feels it is necessary to do everything perfectly. A true desire to do more for a patient can motivate the caregiver to read more and struggle to understand his or her patient better. If, however, the caregiver fears that the slightest error would be catastrophic, the resulting anxiety can be crippling, often leading to care becoming rigid and devoid of the flexibility, individuality, and empathy that caregivers want to provide.

A sense of powerlessness can be equally anxiety provoking and limiting to the caregiver. Frequently a caregiver will experience frustration and inefficiency in specific areas, such as when dealing with other organizations. Too often this experience will become generalized, resulting in a global sense of impotence or incompetence. This "learned helplessness" may then be conveyed to the handicapped person as well, trapping both in a powerless position. If this is recognized, efforts can be made to reappraise the situation and find a more hopeful solution. If, however, hopelessness prevails, true collaborative work becomes very difficult.

Again, the mature caregiver knows that progress in rehabilitation is generally slow and incremental; success is often the result of many small failures along the way. The limitations of the patient's motivation, the institutional bureaucracy, the unexpected setbacks—all at times almost seem as if they were designed to impede and frustrate. But powerlessness and resignation need not be the ultimate end result.

Rigidity is also a common defense against this sense of hopelessness or powerlessness. Finding one particular style or way of doing things, and sticking with that regardless of its appropriateness to the situation, can certainly reduce anxiety, but at a cost. The problem of not knowing what to do is solved, but new problems emerge. The lack of flexibility creates difficulties because patients are so variable in need and response, as in the following situation:

> An 82-year-old man was addressed as "Stan" by his caregivers. This was part of their standard style of casual familiarity with their charges, which they felt created a more "family" atmosphere. However, this man had been a formal, dignified intellectual throughout his life and had *never* been addressed in this way, even by his family. He found it insulting, rather than friendly, and an obstacle to recovery, because it represented a style quite unfamiliar to him. Once this was pointed out, a more workable relationship was negotiated, which helped this man regain most of his previous level of functioning.

A danger for the younger caregiver in interacting with elderly individuals with impairment is to slip into a too-easy familiarity and "chumminess." Younger caregivers may not realize how this reduces the self-respect and pride of a physically compromised senior citizen. It also distorts the reality of the situation. It is best to convey respect for older patients by addressing them by their last name. If that person prefers the first name, he or she will make it clear to the caregiver in subsequent interactions.

## Energy and Anger in the Patient/Caregiver Relationship

Apart from anxiety, anger is the most common response to all stages of body-altering, appearance-altering conditions, whether they be congenital, accidental, or progressive. The caregiver's anger may spring from personal rage at individual recklessness, or perhaps at a capricious God. The focus of the anger may be the patient, who is experienced as argumentative, demanding, hostile, and ungrateful. Other common targets of anger include institutions such as hospitals, rehabilitation centers, or social service networks, which can generally be counted upon to provide multiple sources of frustration and inefficiency. Often these institutional targets are preferred despite the actual source of the anger, because they create less guilt and anxiety for caregivers. Regardless of the source, anger can be overwhelming.

Although many people are uncomfortable with anger, it is both ubiquitous and useful. Despite its potential for destruction, anger can be energizing. Anger organizes one's personality and mobilizes one to take action. It is also appropriate to be angry when agencies or people behave in a biased or inappropriate manner. Experienced caregivers learn that it is neither desirable nor effective to be agreeable at all times. Focused anger can mobilize people to get bills through Congress, and it can push "amputees" to walk. The key is to learn the manner and timing that make most constructive use of the energy of the anger. Some caregivers will deliberately use anger to mobilize depressed patients to fight, increasing independence and energy. Other caregivers will use their own indignation to work in a larger sphere on behalf of the impaired patient. These caregivers have learned how to harness anger to further their work. Unfortunately, caregivers can also be incapacitated by their anger, lashing out at supervisors, peers, or their disabled clients in poorly controlled, and potentially harmful, expressions of their frustration and rage.

A classic example of anger motivating constructive activity is the organization Mothers Against Drunk Driving (MADD), founded by a woman whose son was killed by a drunk driver. Many people find that they can organize and empower themselves for this kind of action to an extent they never felt possible for themselves. This kind of fierce determination can motivate otherwise shy people to speak in public, or help nonassertive individuals to let their needs be known.

Anger can also be used to solidify the alliance between the physically impaired individual and the caregiver. It is common wisdom that an effective way to unite two diverse people or groups is to identify a common enemy. An attitude of "We'll show them!" can provide a basis for energetic and focused work as a team. Sometimes disputes between team members occur over management issues or because of differing styles of relating to each other. These differences can be safely aired in a team meeting as well. Team members can agree to disagree in a way that is not a personal attack on each other. However, sometimes differences cannot be worked out in team meetings, and other arrangements have to be made so that the team can function smoothly. Discussion of these differences often leads to new and creative ways to implement the rehabilitation plan.

## Anxiety and Denial

Caregivers laboring in highly stressful situations need ways to bind the anxiety that is constantly being aroused by the work. Some form of denial is necessary in interacting with people with physical impairment. Although denial is often listed in older psychiatric textbooks as a "primitive" defense, more recent descriptions of denial elevate it to the level of an adaptive response to any powerful trauma. This process, however, usually remains out of our awareness.

Denial is a common response of caregivers, as well as patients, dealing with physical impairments. This may take the form of denial of personal vulnerability (e.g., "Such accidents only happen to wild young athletes, not to sedate professionals like me"), or may extend to a minimization of the patient's own impairment or of its future limitations (e.g., "You may not be able to walk now, but if you do these exercises everyday, you'll be out in the 10K again by next spring").

As with anger, denial can be valuable, if focused and used selectively in moderation. Most of us would never leave our homes if we constantly thought about drive-by shootings or natural disasters. Similarly, to focus optimistically on what one *can* do or *will* do is generally more motivating and useful than to dwell upon what one cannot do. Prophecy can be self-fulfilling. However, it is not helpful to set unattainable goals, which hold no real or partial hope of fulfillment. No useful transaction can be worked between two individuals who are responding to totally separate versions of reality. Acknowledgment of current limitations is essential; focus on these limitations is not. The goal for caregivers is to communicate an empathic understanding of the patient's restrictions, fear, anger, and powerlessness without becoming swept into these feelings and meanings. A bit of denial, like some emotional distancing, can be useful in accomplishing this objective.

The balance between denial and reality is a delicate one for the patient. There are distinct dangers on both sides. Too much denial through unrealistic hope by caregivers in the early stages of a catastrophic injury can impair the patient's facing the magnitude of the injury and doing the coping necessary to deal with it. This in turn can slow the whole rehabilitation process. On the other side, breaking down a patient's denial too quickly so that the patient has no time to bring into operation his or her coping strategies can be equally damaging. Denial (like pain medication) is best titrated to the current level of distress and decreased gradually over time. Big problems can be broken down into their component parts. These smaller problems can then be tackled "head-on" while the larger implications are dealt with gradually. This interchange and titration can best occur in the context of a close, sustained caregiver-patient relationship. Out of that relationship comes moment-to-moment decisions to defer or confront. An example of this was seen with a 10-year-old boy, newly quadriplegic after a neck tumor. The medical staff was disturbed that the boy spoke as though he would someday walk again, something they knew to be impossible. Consultation was needed to help them tolerate the time it took for this young boy to adjust to his loss and slowly accept what his new future held.

In summary, the balance between the patient's recognition of injury and denial of injury is complicated. Caregivers can also err on the other side of this issue by unduly reinforcing denial of the severity of illness and thus prolonging the patient's full recognition of new limitations. This complicated process of titration usually gets worked out in the day-to-day struggles of rehabilitation. It requires the caregiver's full empathic sense as to when to confront, when to support, and when to delay.

## Normal Despair/Normal Hope

Akin to the feelings of helplessness and powerlessness is the despair or hopelessness often experienced by caregivers. It can be difficult to maintain a positive outlook when the activities of the day no longer occupy the mind, or when the support of the team is not always available. Caregivers may experience a visceral sensation of emptiness, loss of energy, even occasional tearfulness, and loss of pleasure in usually enjoyed activities. Some individuals will even notice changes in their eating or sleeping habits. Such mild depressive symptoms can quickly lead to disillusionment with the work, resulting in job changes, or, far worse, caregivers who resent their work and bring no energy or hope to their transactions with their patients. This is what people commonly call "burnout" (Lewiston et al. 1981).

On the other hand, some caregivers leave work at the end of the day uplifted and filled with hope. They find inspiration in the determination and progress of the patients with whom they work. Typically these persons throw themselves into the work and find that the effort expended is directed toward a goal so full of hope that they take home a perspective that improves their general view of the world. They are able to take on other battles with renewed determination and enjoy the successes in their own lives with added zest. This may not be the way they feel *every* day, but this feeling is sufficient to carry them through the inevitable moments of tragedy, frustration, and tedium.

Those who make a career of such work are generally those who can tolerate both these extremes. A disappointment, marking the loss of hope for some specific goal, can be accepted as a part of the process, if later balanced by the sheer joy of another goal finally reached. The lows, while truly low, are not disabling because they are expected, processed, endured, and survived. For example, a therapist working with critically ill children was asked after one death why she kept in the work, since she was obviously saddened by the loss. She reacted with surprise. "I'm sad because I really cared for that child, so I miss him. But if I didn't really care, there would be no point in doing the work. I'd get nothing out of it, and I wouldn't be helpful. When I stop grieving deaths, I'll stop doing this work."

## Search for Meaning

A frequent question posed to caregivers is how they make sense of the suffering, tragedy, and bravery they encounter along the pathway of rehabilitation work. The religious and philosophical questions raised by disabling illness or accidents can be profoundly disturbing and must be dealt with in some way. Often guilt or blame feels more comfortable, for if responsibility can be fixed upon someone, it means the world is still ultimately orderly and under control. Without some sense of orderliness, or meaning, most people feel lost and thus surrender to powerlessness or despair.

Meaning can be found in working with physically impaired people. *Where* an individual finds satisfaction and meaning is dependent upon the caregiver's own personality, beliefs, and background. Some may experience a sense of a "calling" or vocation. Others will see caregiving as a job that perfectly suits their unique skills and interests, or that allows them an opportunity for growth and self-discovery. For most, meaning will be found in the accompaniment of their patients on the metaphorical journey of rehabilitation.

A caregiver must be aware of the tendency to stake too much upon the performance (i.e., the "success" of the work). Meaning must be found in the struggle itself, in the process, not in achieving any particular goals. Objectives are necessary, certainly, but too much must not be invested in particular "destinations." Satisfaction, meaning, and power are inherent in the "journey" and reside within the transaction itself (see Chapter 9). A physical therapist expressed this when she discussed her preference for working with people who had sustained traumatic spinal cord injuries: "If I can inspire even one discouraged young person to strive for optimal independence, all my efforts are worthwhile. It feels so much more meaningful than anything else I could do."

## Summary

How caregivers react to their involvement with those persons who have physical impairments has been the focus of this chapter. Reactions have been described as both intense and far ranging. They can be positive and negative. Courage, determination, and the willingness to make new self-discoveries have been described as some of the ingredients of a successful caregiver. It is an area that brings meaning to the phrase "no pain, no gain." In the next chapter we will discuss ways caregivers can cope with these reactions.

## The Game

You are my friends. You do things
for me. My affliction is
your hangup. It is yours more
than it ever could be mine.
You spread my affliction thin
    enough to go around once
for all of us. You put my
coat on for me when I ask
you. You put my coat on for
me when I do not ask you.
    You embrace my shoes with your
compassion. You tell me I
would be less apt to fall with
rubber soles. You carry things
for me. You tell me they are
    heavy things, how it would be
difficult for anyone
to carry them. You open
mustard bottles for me. You
tell me how hard it is to
    open mustard bottles. I
agree with you. I will not
destroy our game. At night I
dream I am Samson. I will
topple coliseums. I
    will overwhelm you with my
brute power. I will knock you
dead. I will open mustard
bottles for you. I will show
you how easy it really is.

*Harold Bond*

# 6

# Coping Strategies

To this point we have considered the day-to-day transactions between the physically impaired person and the caregiver, with an emphasis on the common and reciprocal but complementary emotional reactions experienced by both. In this chapter we proceed to examine ways in which caregivers and caregiving environments can facilitate coping strategies that are likely to bring about favorable outcomes for patients and staff. Coping (i.e., adaptation to caregiver stresses) will be examined from the perspectives of the individual caregiver, the team, and the institution. The focus is on maintaining balance in a demanding work environment amid complex personal and professional pressures. These same principles may be applicable to volunteers and family members who also function as care providers for persons with physical impairments.

## The Good Caregiver:
## Nurturance as an Ideal

Certain assumptions are often made about what constitutes good coping and good caregiving. The developmental model earlier described (see Chapter 4) parallels the common image of the idealized mother who is nurturant, selfless, and sympathetic. This is the image most of us carry when we are ill or injured. Caregivers often come to expect such ideals of themselves in their interactions with patients, inadvertently omitting a fourth and critical quality of good care, the *ability to set limits,* both on others and on oneself.

Significant risks lurk in following an idealized model of good caregiving. Nurturance and sympathy can easily edge over into infantilization and condescension. *Respect* for the patient requires constant recognition that a need for help does not necessarily imply that someone is helpless or without strengths. Caregivers can become simply dispensers of "good things" with resultant weakening and disenfranchisement of the population served. *Empowering* the patient is based on mutual respect and cooperative work that recognize abilities as well as areas of disability. Consider the following example:

> A 35-year-old attorney was attacked by robbers and left paraplegic. He was angry, angry with everybody. Much of his anger sprang from the powerlessness this previously powerful man was experiencing. Caregivers who tried to soothe him or do things for him quickly learned that he was neither appreciative nor cooperative. It was not until a caregiver challenged him to work on some of the problems himself, to stop feeling sorry for himself and to come up with solutions, that it became possible to use the anger to energize and mobilize this man. At the point of confrontation, the caregiver was not particularly "nice" or nurturant, but approached the patient with both respect and the expectation of capability. This was what was needed for a man struggling with panic in a dependent situation.

The temptation to foster dependency can be subtly pervasive and aided unintentionally by the caregiver and the institution itself. Many caregivers choose their vocation out of a heartfelt and genuine wish to be helpful. The slow pace of rehabilitation work and its inevitable, almost daily disappointments can quickly squash one's self-esteem and leave the caregiver feeling ineffective and diminished. The temptation to demonstrate one's usefulness by fostering dependency in the patient is an understandable response to such frustration. Pity replaces empathy as well-intentioned nurturant impulses begin to place the patient in a lessened position. Broad institutional and political pressures can also subtly push the patient into being more compliant and dependent on hospital routines than is optimal for his or her sense of physical independence or self-determination. Rehabilitation units run too smoothly if patients are not challenged to make decisions for themselves. Sociological studies of hospital procedures have noted that at times procedures appear to be for the convenience of the staff rather than the benefit of the patient (Stubbins 1977; Thomas 1982). A "good hospital" may have a milieu that is somewhat ragged and radiates a sense that there is always something left to be done *by* the patient, not necessarily *for* the patient (Cumming and Cumming 1963). The significance of this issue for patients with physical disabilities who are already threatened by loss of autonomy cannot be overstated. The experienced caregiver will recognize that in some situations when, for example, it would ideally be beneficial to allow patients to feed themselves, it may be necessary for efficiency's sake at certain times to take over, at least temporarily.

Nonetheless, and in spite of individual and institutional frustrations and organizational pressures, many caregivers manage to remain both firm and empathetic, respectful and confident in their work with patients and their colleagues. This is fortuitous but hardly accidental, and the strategies used by these individuals in their work merit specific attention.

## Caring for the Caregivers

Presume for the moment that a major temptation for caregivers who may inadvertently infantilize patients is the caregivers' wish to bolster self-esteem. It follows that primarily empowering caregivers will likely foster a more healthy caregiver self-esteem with subsequent respect for patients. Such respect and power at a staff level can be cultivated by various organizational methods. The *institution* may facilitate or discourage empowerment in its dealings with caregivers. The authority each is given, their benefits, salary, and vacations, and the degree of recognition for specific achievements all speak to the institution's attitude toward its composite staff and endorse in turn the staff's personal sense of professional self-respect. The *unit team* also plays a critical role in caregiver coping. Sharing of difficult tasks, open exchange of advice and criticism, support for difficult decisions, and overall cooperative effort can be done in ways that either support or erode the sense of staff self-respect. Thus, the individual, the team, and the institution, as discussed below, all make significant contributions to the process of successful coping.

### The Individual

Useful coping strategies for the individual are predicated on using the resources of the team and the institution, as will shortly be discussed. Vacations, inservice training opportunities, and educational conferences are only useful if one takes advantage of their availability. The danger is in trying to "do it all." While this may give one a sense of indispensability, over time it is more likely to wear thin and lead to exhaustion, if not burnout. A 15-year veteran nurse put the matter this way:

> When I started out, there wasn't a child here who could be admitted or die without me being there. I was essential, and everybody knew it. It felt good, but I kept getting more exhausted. After about 4 years of that, I just cracked up. Now I make sure other people can do what I do. This

means I can take a vacation or a day off and not get called in. The kids
are still getting good care when I'm not here, and better care when I am,
because I'm not exhausted all the time.

The individual can look to the team and the institution to help
maintain two basic coping techniques: a sense of perspective and a sense
of humor. New caregivers are often startled by the candid and wry
"gallows" humor circulating in a well-established team. Jokes can be
destructive when used as inappropriate put-downs to other caregivers
or patients, but some laughter is essential to keep energy and spirits up
enough to tackle the work. This is especially true in units working with
tough cases or poor-prognosis patients. Some of the most talented
caregivers we have personally known do manage to maintain a ready
sense of "relief-valve" humor. (The humor, of course, is never used to
diminish any patient.)

Discussion of the individual caregiver's occasional needs for psychological assistance for personal problems obviously lies beyond the
scope of this monograph. It remains necessary for caregivers to keep
track of their own feelings in walking the fine line between emotional
release and professional restraint. There are times when a caregiver
simply needs a break, or a different assignment, or a good cry. A sensitive
team member often spots this first, but it is best if caregivers also feel free
to ask for what they need. An institution that permits and encourages
such requests will have happier, more effective employees with lower
rates of turnover and fewer psychological casualties.

Caregivers consistently report that the most rewarding strategy for
coping with job stresses is found in sustained transactions with the
individual patient. Despite the stress involved, most caregivers report
personal fulfillment and professional enrichment sufficient for continuing the task at hand. Long-term line staff report that the satisfaction they
find in the relationships they form with their patients keeps them on the
job (i.e., "at the bedside"). The patient-staff relationship itself also em-
powers some caregivers to advocate for specific change in team or staff
meetings. Such advocacy keeps institutions more closely in touch with
the needs and concerns of its line staff. For caregivers, coping well with
the stresses of their work usually results in more effective coping by the
patients in their charge.

## Local Support: The Team

Most institutions and caregiving facilities are now organized into interdisciplinary teams. As Rothberg (1985) points out, true interdisciplinary

practice is a goal that still does not actually exist in many rehabilitation centers, but one that is worthy of continued pursuit.

Palmer et al. (1985) identified four stages in the development of a multidisciplinary rehabilitation team:

1. **Identification of purpose.** What are the goals for which the team is striving?
2. **Role definition.** Which skills and duties are basic to the functioning of each discipline? Where do the experience and training of each discipline overlap?
3. **Task assignment.** Which tasks are currently performed by each discipline? What are the resources of each discipline in terms of time and personnel?
4. **Integration.** How can the team coordinate the efforts of individual members? How can it educate new members to function well within its structure? What mechanisms does it have in place to reflect on its own functioning? How can consultants contribute to team functioning?

The actual day-to-day functioning of teams varies tremendously by size of institution, range of disciplines represented, and actual decision-making power invested in the team. Nevertheless, most teams are led by a physiatrist and provide two basic functions: 1) an initial treatment plan and 2) a final discharge plan. The team also has many less visible functions.

First, as discussed in the previous chapter, the team can be a common meeting ground for various caregiver expectations. Caregivers can have widely varying expectations for each patient that need to be examined, modified, and coordinated. If one caregiver is expecting a result that other caregivers feel is not realistic, this disparity is sure to be felt by the patient. Likewise, one caregiver's higher expectations may be appropriate, while other caregivers are denying responsibility for these expectations out of fear of the patient's anger. This conflict then becomes an important team issue to resolve.

Second, teams are a safe place to ventilate one's feelings about specific patients as well as about the progress or lack of progress of care. In Chapter 5 we referred to the value of caregivers sharing subjective reactions to patients with other caregivers in gaining insight about both patients and themselves. The team is a crucial arena in which to buffer and modify these often intense reactions. If not dealt with openly, negative feelings can influence the team collectively to "punish" or scapegoat certain patients without quite being aware of what they are doing (Graves 1978; Mullins 1989). Some teams anticipate this situation by having regularly scheduled consultation with a mental health consultant. This allows a more reflective interchange to occur and encourages more in-depth review of the team process. These reactions can then be translated into strategies of care that are more consistent and beneficial. A climate of trust and confidentiality are obvious prerequisites for such sharing.

Another mechanism for handling the buildup of frustration and developing new patterns of interaction is a team *retreat*. It is important to define the purpose of such retreats carefully so that they are not mistaken for group therapy. The boundaries between self-revelation and work-group recognitions can be tricky and are important to respect. The assistance of an experienced mental health consultant to help process the issues and the needs of the group appropriately without allowing the discussion to spill over into therapeutic issues of particular individuals is needed. Team maintenance and task performance are the goal of such discussions.

A team faces a number of dilemmas. A team can easily overwhelm a struggling patient's need for autonomy during rehabilitation with their collective need to "call the shots" (Purtillo 1988). This form of paternalism may work against the patient's sense of investment in the treatment goals. On the other hand, teams may have to go against a patient's particular wishes at times in order promote the patient's best interest. When patient and team clash over ways of doing things, it is important to recognize that the patient can feel overwhelmed in such a conflict and may retreat into a stance of passive hostility that works against the long-term goals of rehabilitation that the team is supporting. There is no easy solution to such a dilemma, but it is important that the team not become a closed system, resistant to change. A sense of openness and a willingness to reflect on one's collective behavior are crucial.

Teams need to develop ways of welcoming new members (as well as new ideas) that provide for team continuity and at the same time foster a sense of belonging to each new participant. Each new member is eager to be useful and to have a particular role to play. The more quickly that happens, the more secure that new team member will be. Similarly, rituals are needed for those leaving the team so that a sense of closure occurs for the remaining team members. The way a team shows appreciation for the departing person demonstrates to all involved the value given to each on the team.

Teams serve clinical needs rather than administrative needs. Beyond the team, each caregiver is part of the larger ethos that comprises the institution. Good administrative structure and function, as discussed below, are no less vital to good patient care than is the team.

## The Institution: A Framework of Support

Institutions, of necessity, are run by administrators who carry out the policies, priorities, and values of their particular organization. Each organization provides a central frame of support and encouragement for caregiver efforts, signaled most directly by salary and direct benefits. Caught between third-party payers and the rightful demands of the line staff, the hospital communicates its approval with the salary schedule it provides staff. But the institution also conveys the value it places on its staff in many other, less tangible ways as well.

**Authorization.** Recently a public airline emphasized its policy authorizing each flight attendant to make decisions in the interest of its customers that would be automatically backed by the administration. The importance of such a policy is not only the circumventing of cumbersome bureaucratic tangles, but the shifting of focus to the immediate person at hand in solving a problem, rather than forcing the customer to run a corporate maze. A worker thus empowered, at whatever level, feels less confined and more trusted and is therefore more likely to be truly invested in the transaction itself. For such a process to work, the institution must of course give credibility to such a stand. The authorization must be clear and must not exceed the capacity of the employee.

For example, authority for hospital discharge planning can be delegated to a professional who is adequately trained and suitably equipped for the task. That person would have access to appropriate resources with a set of general guidelines. Excessive rigidity in guidelines imperils the need to make an individualized, creative plan for each patient. On the other hand, authorizations that exceed the abilities of the caregiver can be just as detrimental to good patient care. Care providers should be able to make discharge planning decisions with medical backup and with a sense of responsibility and self-confidence that is in line with their skill level.

**Benefits and perquisites.** Institutional recognition of job difficulty or skill level is typically salary related. However, in many settings a combination of benefits, leave time, schedule flexibility, and communal pride is sufficient to retain fulfilled and productive staff against a financial gradient. These benefits (beyond insurance) include staff lounges, social gatherings, child care, improved work settings, access to housing, access to clubs and organizations, and funding for continuing education. These can often be of more *real* value to an employee than extra salary. The number of hours worked is frequently less important than *when* these hours are worked. Flexible hours and child care often mark the critical difference between a happy, relaxed worker and a chronically tired, harassed, and embittered one. Leave times likewise are not measured solely in terms of days but also in flexibility and coverage provided. Taking 2 weeks of vacation when no one else wants to go, and during which work accumulates and messages go unanswered, can feel more frustrating and exhausting than the "vacation" is worth. Frequent genuine opportunities to be recharged, refreshed, and revitalized are necessary to maintain the emotional and professional energy necessary for providing good care.

For such flexible coverage and vacations to work, there must be smooth cooperation and suitable planning within the system. A sense of community, established at an institutional level within the work environment, fosters the team sense that allows people to work cooperatively. If workers feel *their* needs are respected, they can then look after the needs of others in a similar manner and with similar respect. Pride in the institution and its work is a powerful incentive and reward for a caregiver *if* the individual feels like a participant in that overall organization. If no opportunity for input or respect is available, the caregiver gradually feels frustration and bitterness. High staff turnover is the eventual result.

**Acknowledgment of needs and recognition of achievement.**    In any work setting the caregivers with the most direct care responsibilities tend to be those with the least formal education. They tend to receive the lowest pay and occupy the lowest position in the staff hierarchy (Keith 1988). It is critically important to find appropriate ways of recognizing the work of frontline people, whose general contributions can be easily overlooked. Communication of respect for the work such staff do must be consciously planned so that it becomes normative to recognize, rather than to assume, such important effort. Recognition is also important for those individuals who have special needs and for those who have performed an exceptional task or accomplishment. A caregiver who has surmounted a personal or professional obstacle, who has solved a sticky and troublesome problem, or who has achieved advanced education or demonstrated unusual competence, deserves specific recognition from the parent organization.

Institutions must also acknowledge that some situations require unusual arrangements in order to provide care for their own staff. For example, one caregiver in a facility for neurologically impaired adults had been repeatedly threatened (while others had not been) by a particular patient. Rather than risk a permanent loss of confidence and ability of this individual to deliver direct care, the unit chief reassigned this person to another area until she could rebuild her shaken confidence and develop strategies to comfortably reenter the primary care situation.

The reader will notice the interconnectedness among each set of activities. Good patient care will be affected by the bedside relationship with caregivers. These relationships, in turn, will be affected by what occurs at the team meeting. The team functioning will be affected by the values espoused and by the organizational structure of the institution itself. All these factors are needed and all are vital as each patient continues the journey of rehabilitation.

Strategies of caregiver coping are also closely intertwined with the actual transactions that occur between caregiver and patient. Our attention now shifts to these transactions.

## Rehabilitation Center

In the good suburb, in the bursting season,
their canes sway in the yellow day,
the newly maimed mince back to danger.

Cave by cave they come to build their hearing
hard as fists against the jangling birds,
the slipslop of car wheels, walls' mimicries,

the hollow rebuttal of planes. Curbs curse them.
Puddles damn their simplicity. At lot lines
forsythia is a swipe across the face.

Under a wide sky let them cry now
to be coddled, misread a tree, black shins,
or crack their knees on countermands;

the downgrade is uncertain for us all.

In time they will grow competent,
love us, test and correct, feel words
on their quiet skin, begin to light our lamps.

Six weeks and they will swing around these corners,
grotesque and right, their appetites restored.
It is true the sun is only heat,

but distance, depth, doorsills
are ridged on their maps until
they know exactly where they are now.

I see their lockstep right as lilac buds.

*Maxine Kumin*

# 7

# Therapeutic Transactions

## Simple Acts, Complex Interactions

On the journey of rehabilitation, the day-to-day transactions that occur between caregiver and patient often have a routine and rather ritualized quality. Getting the paraplegic patient into his or her wheelchair and off to occupational therapy; assisting in the daily dressing changes of a burned patient—all such daily acts can be done almost without thinking much about their significance. But all such simple acts have the potential to be therapeutic transactions as well. By "therapeutic" we mean the potential to bring about some healing in the broadest sense of that term. Most of us can think of individuals who make life a little easier in moment-to-moment or day-to-day professional activities. Sometimes seemingly simple acts between caregiver and patient can have considerable meaning for both. These acts provide a kind of gentle lubrication that makes hospitals or care facilities more tolerable and humane.

An illustration of this notion comes easily to mind. We know an elevator operator at a rehabilitation institute who does informal "therapy" all day long but would be shocked to ever hear it called such. This individual has worked at the institute for 25 years and thus knows everyone quite well. He has an uncanny sense of knowing when to be humorous and when to be serious. There are times when he has been known even to be gently confrontational. Both patients and caregivers seem to feel just a bit better when they get off this elevator than when they got on. If one asked him whether he knew how important his therapeutic role was, he would deny it with the same good nature with which he greets people. Hospitals, rehabilitation centers, and clinics all have special people of this sort who use the daily rituals of care to bring about small acts of healing. Of course, there are certain times when the patient and the caregiver interact in a much more intense and sustained way. A wide variety of such transactions will be addressed as we focus on these interchanges in the setting of the rehabilitation center.

In the odyssey of rehabilitation, staff and patients become reciprocally bound together through actions, ideas, and feelings. Nowhere is this reciprocity more vivid than in the phase of active institutionally based rehabilitation. The rehabilitation setting places a particularly heavy emotional burden on patients and families. Why should this be so?

Rehabilitation and convalescence represent an experience of dramatic conflicting change for patients. In the acute phase of hospital treatment, patients become accommodated to a forced dependent state in which they renounce most responsibility for themselves and submit to the authority of physician and nurse. In exchange, there is an expectation that the treatments will (as if by magic) restore them to preillness normalcy. Those persons experiencing nonfatal, life-threatening, life-altering catastrophic illness discover that although they are no longer acutely "ill," they are still far from being "cured" or returned to a truly normal state. If not "cured," then what solace is available for persons in a "twilight zone," who are yet unable to resume a life of optimal activity and independence? Rehabilitation is a form of treatment in which the goal is the restoration of maximal functioning, not cure. Adapting to this change in self-expectation involves a type of painfully upsetting psychological work analogous to the well-known "grief work" of a bereaved person's struggle with the loss of a loved one (as mentioned in Chapter 3).

## Caregivers, Individual Patients, and the System

Patients usually begin their rehabilitation without a sense of what is in store for them. The loss of previous bodily function needs to be acknowledged. If patients have spent time in a hospital, they most likely have retained residues of the hospital role: obedience to hospital order and expectant waiting for restoration to normalcy. For the rehabilitation experience to be effective, the patient's role must change to that of an active, rather than passive, participant in daily activities as well as overarching social and vocational decisions. Of necessity there is a vast amount of trial-and-error behavior, false starts, unavoidable disagreements, and conflicts as patient and caregivers learn a mutually acceptable and workable "common language" of transactional relationship. It is such a relationship that in turn becomes the vehicle for sound and effective rehabilitation. Several basic transactional principles that often occur in the context of this journey through the rehabilitation center are described below.

First, some distress is a sign of life and health. This distress is likely to occur in both caregiver and patient. The price a dedicated caregiver pays for his or her constructive involvement with patients with physical impairments is that he or she will periodically become emotionally upset by the transactional work. If the caregiver is not occasionally upset, there is probably not any significant interpersonal involvement. The professional working with severely damaged persons learns several protective caveats:

1. It is generally helpful to stay in contact with one's own emotional reactions regarding a patient or illness.
2. It is helpful to recognize the universality of those feelings as they occur in other sensitive and sensible caregivers.
3. It is critical to manage such feelings in the service of patient care *so that neither patient nor caregiver suffers adverse consequences as a result of the interaction.*

Recall here our initial premise that patients tend to move along developmental pathways from initial forced regression to progressive autonomy and independence (see Chapter 4). Along this pathway patients go through experiences in which they express painful feelings by lashing out at themselves, at the caregivers, and at the world in ways that we normally do not allow ourselves. Eventually such permission has to be modified as the patient moves through the process of rehabilitation and can handle larger amounts of frustration. As the patient learns to tolerate more frustration without erupting, so the caregiver (in parallel fashion) learns to manage his or her subjective distress in ways that do not interfere directly with patient care.

A second premise is that conflicted transactions in rehabilitation work usually occur at the interface of two "systems" (patient/staff, staff/family, clinical/administrative, etc.). It is at these interfaces that failures to communicate and empathize most often occur. Such conflicts can gain momentum and become more total failures in rehabilitation if not recognized and resolved with dispatch.

Examples of this interface conflict are numerous (also see Chapter 10):

- A patient and nurse are at a standoff over the (depressed) patient's refusal to get up and begin the complex task of dressing before scheduled therapy.
- A physician angrily demands to know why the physical therapist has been unable to carry out the ordered treatment, not accepting the answer "Simply because the patient was unwilling."

- The team confronts the social worker with the task of getting an intrusive mother to have more appropriate and productive interactions with the staff.
- The team presents the psychiatric consultant with the task of motivating the disorganized patient into cooperative (compliant) behavior.

It is at the interface between systems that delays, miscommunications, irritations, misinterpretations, and ultimately treatment/disposition errors may occur, leaving everyone unhappy and prone to blame others for the problems.

A third premise is again based on the notion that caregiver and patient are part(s) of a system, and that over time what is good for resolving the patient's problems will be in the ultimate best interests of the caregiver as well. For instance, fostering a patient's autonomy not only is important for the patient's future capacity to live independently once hospitalization is over, but it also serves as a constructive check on the caregiver's tendency to be autocratic or authoritarian. Similarly, as team members spend time together attending to their own collective emotional understanding of the patients in their care, patients' needs will then be attended to in a more sophisticated, integrated, and empathic manner. The mental health of both patient and caregiver can be enhanced by some reflective time away from the bedside to explore some of the more concealed communications of each patient.

We recognize that a therapeutic transaction cannot be easily scheduled or "packaged." It is the regular caregiver who is responsible for moment-to-moment and day-to-day care who will be the likely agent of therapy regardless of job title or rank. We recall the housekeeper at a major academic center who was once asked to give a grand rounds presentation on her ability and methods of cheering up oncology patients! The presentation was heartfelt and sincere. The principle that most "psychological" issues will be handled by those most in contact with the person was thus clearly and publicly substantiated. Any clinician can testify to the critical quality of the abilities and personality of the ward secretary in the day-to-day operations of a clinical unit.

It is safe to say that the patient will share the strongest feelings with (and be the most responsive to) the person with whom he or she feels safest. Again, that "safe" person is the caregiver most in attendance and most visible to the patient, not necessarily the one highest in the medical hierarchy. Physicians are generally less immediately available in ward routine and yet hold more authority and thus may not be the "safest" for sharing critical emotions and issues. This issue is another reason why team meetings are crucial to efficient and effective care. Information about the patient that is central to good care and progress may only be made known through line staff. That information may be crucial in the team's obtaining an optimal understanding of the patient.

## Confirming Techniques in Common Acts

From these several general statements about transactions in a rehabilitation setting, more specific suggestions are now offered. The assumption is made that every patient has a healthy adult "self" that will be able to process these interventions in an appropriate manner. At the risk of sounding a bit didactic, some specific admonitions are listed:

1. **Listen!** It is impossible to overemphasize the enhancement of a patient's self-esteem that comes through the caregiver's "simply listening" seriously and respectfully. It might even seem trite to mention such an ordinary human response, yet the simplest things are easily overlooked in a busy institution. There are frequent instances when the most valuable things we can do *for* a patient is to give that person some of our valuable time, instead of rushing off to our next pressing duty. Why is this so? It conveys firmly and immediately that we think (and act as though we believe) that the person is important enough to listen to. In so doing, we automatically convey some sense of the value we attach to the person and our respect for the patient as an equal human being. One sits (not stands) alongside the patient and attends to the patient's comments of the moment. Not only does listening convey respect, it also is very supportive. Both the patient and the patient's family need more chances to talk to caregivers than they often get. Because listening consumes time, it is "experience," particularly for the health professional with wide areas of responsibility. But listening also requires us to deal with our own responses to what is said. This takes emotional energy on the part of caregivers. What one hears, as Dr. William Carlos Williams said (see Chapter 4), is often so stirring that "you get stopped in your tracks by something the patient says, and it takes time to let its way through your head and heart."
2. **Accept.** The validity of the patient's comments is acknowledged as a first step toward separating the patient from consequent obligatory behavior. "Yes, if I were paralyzed from the neck down, I too might feel like ending my life. But I don't always act on every feeling." Granting validity provides opportunity for tempering and temporizing the affect of the moment into a more thoughtful, balanced view of the situation, and it also relieves some anxiety for the patient.

3. **Negotiate.** A variety of tools exist to assist patients in their movement from maladaptive (generally "frozen") positions to more flexible stances. A graded series of negotiations can assist movement, from the rational/logical down through maneuvers of convincing, coaxing, cajoling, and (if necessary) coercion. "If you come out of your cocoon of the bedclothes and go to your two most important therapies, I'll let you skip the others, but for this week only." Occasionally honest "bribery" is acceptable when it is subservient to the treatment goals and conducted within an open and acknowledged framework of support.

4. **Support.** Endorsing both the past and the present abilities of the patient appeals to his or her normal but latent self-esteem and can be a powerful form of gentle persuasion. "How can a woman as bright as you've been all your life, and with these accomplishments, now be acting so shortsightedly and counterproductively?" Taking caution not to dichotomize the current disability, and tapping reservoirs of esteem (always available in any patient's personal history), one can provide support for the moment and serve in the long run to weave past and future lives together by bridging catastrophic change with threads of common experience.

5. **Reward.** Firm and honest admiration for goals well accomplished (however small) shifts individuals in the direction of future accomplishments. Requiring no insight or introspection on the part of the patient, strict behavioral feedback can accomplish therapeutic responses in the most resistant of clients. "Knowing as I do how upsetting it is for you to be seen in public when you feel so disfigured, I'm very impressed that you have the courage to eat in a hospital cafeteria and even to go out on a field trip." The patient does not need to endorse the insights to gain strength from the comment.

6. **Forgive.** Short-term retreats, such as temporary removal from excessive stimulation or staff pressure to improve, allow a disorganized or overwhelmed patient to take a break and "reintegrate." "We're going to let you spend a day in a quiet room, curtains drawn, and if necessary with a sitter. Everybody has days when they get so frightened and upset that it's impossible to do any kind of decent work. But tomorrow I think you'll be much better, and we can resume your rehabilitation activities." Central to this approach is backing off, acknowledging regression, avoiding blame or coercion, and then, regrouping, pressing on to the necessary tasks. This principle is inherent in respite care programs, inpatient psychiatry units, and everyday life (e.g., weekends, vacations, retreats). It is critical that one not get so enthused for the work at hand (often with a fire fanned by third-party payers or rehabilitation goals) that one forgets to back

off when the patient is perilously vulnerable and "try again in the morning."

7. **Set firm (but progressive) limits.** Firm limit setting with respect to out-of-control behavior combined with an explicit promise not to abandon the patient can ensure a persistent positive direction. "Your difficult behavior upsets us, but it's your behavior, not you, that we are angry at. And if you think that behavior like that will drive us to throw you out or abandon your program, you're dead wrong. So just stop the nonsense. We know you can do better." Inherent in any therapy, the principle of tolerating (but limiting) the bad while ferreting out and encouraging the good seems equally useful in the rehabilitation setting. The art is in both the timing and the balance. One must judge when the patient can "hear" such a message.

## The Darker Side: Caveats and Pitfalls

None of us always say the right thing at the right time. Parents can recall the (frequent) times their responses to their children were less than mature, and yet somehow most children learn to sense the intent as well as the words. So it is with professional caregiving roles. One can often be caught off guard by the unexpected outburst or demand. Some days we are plain tired and do not have the energy to process the messages we receive in a mature fashion. All of us can recall times when we responded to our patients in a less than desirable fashion. What follows is a listing of specific interventions (here of the negative variety) with examples:

1. **Coercion.** Threats to abandon or punish the patient in an either/or context are rarely necessary. "Stop that behavior or we'll call the psychiatrist. Keep it up and we'll discharge you." The either/or context "boxes" the patient (and caregiver) into adversarial emotional corners and usually escalates, rather than resolves, the conflict. Open exploration of the disagreement becomes impossible. Introducing psychiatry as punishment impedes the value of a subsequent consultation.

2. **Invoking guilt.** Efforts to control or manipulate a patient by working on guilt rarely prove productive over the long run. "You're being a bad parent by not wanting to get on with the program. Think of what you owe your family!" Guilt is a poor motivator in the long run, either in family dynamics or in the medical care setting. One can fairly assume that regressed patients are already enormously guilty by virtue of their enforced dependence on others. More guilt usually drives the patient in the opposite direction from that intended.

3. **Hollow exhortation.** Efforts at arm twisting rarely produce sustained benefits and often reveal as much (or more) about the internal dynamics and family background of the twister than either the caregiver or the surrounding staff may wish to examine. "Forget about being depressed. Hard work will help you feel better." Moralistic appeals rarely benefit the patient, although they have the surface appeal of being a significant "intervention." A simple reflecting back to the patient of the dilemma may have more impact. "You feel so down now, it doesn't seem like you'll ever want to try again. But I think you will." The same applies to the often-heard, "It could have been worse." Only the *patient* has the right to that statement as injury and loss are reviewed and "processed" in the grieving itself. Such a response may prevent the patient from coming to grips with the range and extent of the injury. It also may prolong the patient's unrealistic denial about what has happened.

   A false exhortation can come in many more subtle forms as well. Consider the following example.

   > An elderly woman recovering from a stroke complained to her husband that the "encouragement" she was receiving from her physical therapist was getting on her nerves. Everything she did was "great." "You're doing beautifully, Virginia!" was simply not the case, and this woman knew it. She felt the condescension contained in this repetitive bit of false encouragement.

   Caregivers have to guard against a kind of mechanistic, unfeeling praise that can unthinkingly become a part of one's repertoire but may not be appreciated by every patient.

4. **Overindulgence (fostering dependency).** Every caregiver has an idea of an appropriate response to a patient's inappropriate request. The underlying assumption probably is that patients could do the acts themselves, or that perhaps they should not have the wish in the first place, let alone expect anyone to satisfy it. Overindulgence in meeting these requests has two potential hazards: 1) it turns patients away from learning to maximize autonomous behavior, and 2) it foments childishly arrogant ideas of power that can be frightening to patient and staff. "All I have to do is demand and threaten, and my caregivers will jump to meet my demands, as if by the magical power of my voice." The task is to evaluate the patient's request in the context of the total rehabilitation progress and goals. This is never easy to do. Sometimes a bit of humor lubricates the interaction with the patient who makes inappropriate demands, but humor must be used with care as well.

5. **Competition.** Competitive control can arise in a variety of arenas, including simple daily care, family dynamics, pace of progress, or goals of treatment. Our own painful reactions to catastrophically damaged and subsequently disabled patients can threaten us and make us uncertain about our abilities to be helpful, or even significant. "There but for the grace of God go I" is simultaneously a philosophical condolence (for the caregiver) and a subtly competitive self-serving detachment, implying both superiority of position and divine favoritism. Our identification with our patient, allowing as it does the constructive possibility of empathy and involvement, also confronts us with our feared frailties and vulnerability. The patient is damaged and we are (temporarily) intact, and, philosophical arguments to the side, it is critical that we not take a stance beside the patient predicated on this unspoken hierarchy of function. Such feelings are ubiquitous and must be acknowledged and dealt with honestly (and at times openly) to remain effectively engaged in such work. Here, perhaps more than in any other area of intervention, the professional and personal agendas of the caregiver must be subject to continued scrutiny and kept as clear as possible.

## Exculpation and Benediction

Finally, it is important to remind our reader (and ourselves) that one can never be quite sure whether any particular transaction has been all that helpful or all that harmful. Even if we say or do the "right thing," our patient may not give us some form of confirming feedback. Over the long phase of the rehabilitation journey, it is our attitude rather than any particular words that carries the most impact. If we can demonstrate an openness about the fact that we "goof," that we sometimes make mistakes, that in the long run our outcomes are imperfect, then we model an attitude useful for patients to adopt as well. Caregivers persist in the struggle, maintain positive motivation in spite of inevitable failures, and accommodate amicably to suboptimal results on a day-to-day basis.

In the rehabilitation care system, every caregiver is a teacher of sorts, and every caregiver is also a therapist. Caregivers can be effective in their interventions if they recognize that these tasks carry special meanings. The meaning of what is said or how it is said may not be immediately clear to the patient or caregiver. Sometimes only time or further reflection clarifies the significance of any particular interaction. The possibility of new understandings, strengths, and commitments makes the work of each caregiver pleasurable and satisfying. It also aids in the healing process that occurs during rehabilitation.

The first reaction a normal individual or good-legger has is, "Oh gee, there's a fellow in a wheelchair," or "There's a fellow with a brace." And they don't say, "Oh gee, there's so and so, he's handsome," or "he's intelligent," or "he's a bore," or what have you. And then as the relationship develops they don't see the handicap. It doesn't exist anymore. And that's the point that you as a handicapped individual become sensitive to. You know after talking with someone for a while when they don't see the handicap anymore. That's when you've broken through.

*Fred Davis*[1]

---

[1]Davis F: "Deviance disavowal: the management of strained interaction by the visibly handicapped," in *The Other Side*. Edited by Becker HS. New York, Free Press, 1964, p. 123.

# 8

# Community Living:
# The Final Destination

A return to living in the community is for most people with physical impairment their ultimate destination on the journey back. This chapter is composed of two major sections. In the first section we detail the return of the patient from an inpatient setting to the community. Such an examination starts with a brief history of caregiving throughout the ages and also looks at the epidemiology of people with physical impairments living in the United States. Transitional issues are then spelled out in some detail. Pressures in the family and the workplace as they influence the returning individual are discussed. This is followed by a look at the issue of common social attitudes toward those persons with physical impairment.

In the second section of this chapter we discuss the role of the caregiver in the community. Special issues germane to caregiving in a community setting are spelled out, as are particular forms of intervention appropriate to community life.

## Returning to the Community

### A Brief History of Caregiving

As long as civilization has existed, some forms of caregiving have also existed. The care of a parent for a child is the most basic form this process takes and, of course, is essential to the survival of the human race. There is an old Russian proverb in which it is said that you cannot pay someone to do what a mother will do for free. Yet caregiving for those with pronounced physical impairment usually moves beyond an intrafamily context and is affected by attitudes of the entire society. Caregiving in this context gains a professional status; it is sanctioned by societal values that in turn are communicated through those institutions that society constructs for this purpose. Unfortunately social acceptance of physical disability has been slower to come than have advances in medical care. The alteration of one's body by a physical impairment invariably changes one's relationship to society. Joseph Newman (1983) points out that societies have treated their physically disabled members according to the current philosophy of their age and time. He detects over the course of history three main societal attitudes toward the physically impaired. All three remain today.

First, an attitude of utilitarianism has at times predominated. This notion means that one's usefulness to society is the major criterion of one's value. Thus, in primitive societies, diseased and disabled persons were sometimes seen as burdens to the group. Children and the aged were also viewed in a similar fashion, particularly during hard times. Individuals in all these groups could be periodically killed or abandoned. Now such practices seem harsh and cruel, but at the time they were considered necessary for survival. For instance, in Europe during the Middle Ages, children with birth defects were called "changelings." They were believed to be the offspring of a woman's union with the devil. A woman suspected of practicing witchcraft would be asked if she had given birth to a changeling, and an admission could result in burning at the stake (Hoffter 1968).

Second, with the advent of the Renaissance, the emergence of humanitarianism toward persons with handicaps could be discerned. Human life in all its forms was emphasized as sacred, and compassion was stressed as a moral force. People like St. Vincent de Paul established homes for abandoned children and hospices for chronically ill persons. Even so, Christianity still saw disease and disability as the scourge of God, as punishment for sin, or as discipline to be endured (Apt 1965). Moral writings have often linked physical perfection with moral superiority and physical "blemish" with spiritual deficit. For instance, until well into this century the United States census counted disabled people with willful criminals as one class (Darling 1982). Both were considered deviant.

Lastly, the third philosophy guiding society's treatment of the handicapped, the concept of *rights,* is based directly upon law. In this country, specifically in the Constitution and the Bill of Rights, these rights are contained in the Fifth and Fourteenth Amendments. This third movement goes beyond humanitarianism in its insistence that individuals exercise active roles in reaching decisions on matters that affect them. The movement to gain these rights for people with disabilities began in the 1950s and developed rapidly in the ensuing years, culminating in legislation enacted in the 1970s in which the rights of disabled persons to protection against discrimination and other forms of unjust treatment were further elaborated (Newman 1983).

These three philosophies interact concurrently in present day endeavors and proposals to initiate and guide plans for physically impaired people. As an example, the utilitarian approach has always exerted a powerful influence on legislators in arguing that disabled people can become productive taxpayers. Deinstitutionalization in the 1970s was fueled by its promise to reduce mounting costs of operating large institutions. Thus no matter how desirable a "legislative goal," such as government services for the physically impaired (i.e., humanitarianism), it should also be "cost effective" (i.e., utilitarian) (Newman 1983).

This brief description of seeming historical progress does not capture the power of social stigma on a personal level. As individuals, we never meet the sociological abstraction "society." What we do encounter are other individuals, and it is through such meetings that we build an image of society, of how we relate to it, and of where we stand within it. So it is with those who have disabilities. Whatever the current rhetoric, physically disabled people are still seen as "the problem," and comparatively little attention is paid to the ways in which society forces them into an inferior role, preventing their access to a wide range of amenities and limiting their opportunities. Still deeply embedded are societal attitudes of charity and condescension (Thomas 1982). The visibly disabled person is customarily accorded "surface acceptance, like the poor man at the wedding; sufficient that he is here but he should not expect to dance with the bride" (Davis 1964, p. 128).

## The Epidemiology of Physical Impairment in the United States

It is easier to determine the prevalence of heart disease or cancer than the prevalence of physical impairments, because currently there is no universally accepted definition of either the process or the taxonomy of disability. Most data about impairments, disabilities, and handicaps are collected by agencies interested in specific information only. Nevertheless, rough estimates have been made. The best overview of impairments, disabilities, and handicaps in the United States was developed by the U.S. Commission on Civil Rights in 1983. Their guess is that about 43 million Americans have some form of impairment, disability, or handicap (Hahn 1983). This figure includes chronic health conditions, work limitations, educational limitations, and transportation handicaps.

Conservative estimates are that between 10% and 20% of children in America experience some long-term illness and that 2% to 4% of children have severe health conditions that affect their daily lives on a regular basis (Perrin and MacLean 1988). Around 10% of adults in the United States have some form of work disability. Between 6% and 9% of school children receive some form of special education, particularly speech and learning assistance. There is a greater chance of being disabled the older one gets. If one is of minority status, the rate of disabilities also goes up (8% of whites are considered disabled compared with 13% of blacks and 13% of Hispanics). Only 25% of the disabled receive some form of rehabilitation. Individuals receiving rehabilitative services primarily have musculoskeletal, developmental, or sensory disabilities. Impairments, disabilities, and handicaps also affect one's economic productivity. A disabled person on the average earns only a quarter of the income of the nondisabled person. Only 40% of disabled persons work. Those severely disabled who work tend to do so on the average of less than 40 hours per week.

## Moving Back to the Community

This transition to the community can be a wrenching experience. Despite the careful anticipation and instruction given by caregivers in hospital and rehabilitation settings, the return home is not easy. For as demanding as the activities of the rehabilitation experience were, there was a certain stability and predictability that is now gone. Support was provided and aims were clearly defined. Food and shelter were taken for granted. The "real" world in the community offers much less structure and more uncertainty. To a returning person with a physical impairment, the world can look very impersonal; it is filled with unpredictable expectations and vastly restricted opportunities for self-fulfillment. But above all, the need to build new relationships, many of which have to be constructed (or reconstructed) from scratch, is the most imposing task.

When discharged, persons with physical impairment face something that they will have had very little opportunity to experience when hospitalized: a world that is not particularly well accommodated to their new status nor motivated to meeting them even halfway (Thomas 1982). They will face architectural and transportation barriers and a multiplicity of job and educational obstacles. Instead of an integrated, need-oriented health care system, these persons will face a health care delivery system comprised of separate units, each oriented toward delivering its own restricted service in its own idiosyncratic way. They will face the task of managing their activities of daily living without many of the special environmental alterations and selective assistance that had been available in the rehabilitation unit. They will face stigma in the form of society's anxiety-based or ignorance-based contempt, indifference, or outright condemnation.

In this chapter the exploration of the special burdens, both psychological and situational, faced by physically impaired persons returning to the community will be followed by the ways in which the caregiver's relationship to these burdens produces a different set of psychological issues for caregivers.

The interactions in the community between caregiver and former patient, although different, are no less complex than those in a hospital or rehabilitation center, and opportunities for satisfaction or frustration in each participant abound.

To introduce these issues in the return to the community for someone with a major physical impairment, five vignettes are offered. Each illustrates a significant challenge for both former patients and their caregivers.

**The ordeal of the transition.**    Jack Hofsiss, in an interview with Jean Smith and George Plimpton (1989), gives a poignant example of the difficulties in moving from institution to home:

> Mr. Hofsiss had at the age of 28 won a Tony award for his direction of "The Elephant Man." Just 6 years later, in 1985, a near-fatal swimming pool accident that fractured his spine left him paralyzed from the chest down. At the time the accident occurred, his career was so successful that he had begun to think, "With a great sense of hubris, that there was no limit to my horizons." This contrasted sharply with the long and grueling recuperation that followed the accident. As Mr. Hofsiss reported:
>
> > *The hardest part of the journey for me was returning home* [emphasis added]. When you're in the hospital, its anonymity allows you to keep at a distance the fact that your life has been unalterably changed and played with. When you get home, you're around all the things in your daily life that you had the year before when you could walk yourself into the kitchen, get yourself a cup of coffee or a glass of milk. That's where the serious adjusting takes place.
>
> Mr. Hofsiss went through a period of depression, a profound sense of loss of self, and a recurring preoccupation with ending his life. The beginning of his recovery came with the encouragement he received to take up his profession again, despite the impairment.

Hofsiss found that his relationship with theater had changed and that his involvement had become much more profound. He began to appreciate the process of creating as more important than the product created (i.e., success). He was one of those physically impaired individuals who was fortunate enough to be able to return to his original work role. But all the working through to the point of reestablishing his new role and new self took considerable time and great effort.

**The family ordeal.**    It is not the patient alone upon whom falls the burden of adjustment to community living. There are severe injuries that leave little or no cosmetic clue or trace; yet the resulting disability is great, and the stress on the affected family can be cumulative and unrelenting (Urbach and Culbert 1991). An obvious example is that of a young person who sustains a closed head injury:

> A 19-year-old college freshman had received a severe brain contusion in a car accident. She had been comatose for a week, then began an arduous rehabilitation program. Two months later she returned home, but not with her former abilities. She now had the intellectual and social skills of a preadolescent child in the body of a young adult woman. By appearance, she seemed normal, until she spoke or tried to do something age appropriate. The family had put their own plans to move "on hold" while they marshalled their energies toward obtaining special educational services that this young woman required. They had to be constantly on guard lest she wander away from the home unprotected. Even while they were managing this "new" person in their midst, the family had to work through the grief they felt for having lost their normal child. The issue of establishing a new emotional equilibrium in this family is formidable indeed.

An entirely different set of problems face the family in which an elderly person returns home after, for example, a stroke or a hip fracture. Is this person able to be self-sufficient? Provisions for home care require an enormous amount of planning during the hospital or rehabilitation stay so that the transition can occur relatively smoothly, as in the following example:

> A 72-year-old bachelor recovering from open-heart surgery had a prior history of alcoholism and was recently found to have diabetes. Both his family and the attending physician felt he should move to a nursing home. He was adamantly against this and insisted on returning to his modest dwelling in a remote rural area. Over a 4-month period of frequent weekend visits from staff at the Veterans Administration hospital, he was able to convince the medical staff that he was capable of handling himself at home.

He has biweekly visits from a visiting nurse as well as regular visits from a nephew and cousin. So far, so good. But each situation is complex and must be considered individually.

**The threat of change.** Even when a relatively stable community adjustment has been achieved at considerable cost, each new change is a painful reminder of one's limitation. Even with a minor change, the whole anxiety-ridden process of relearning and readjustment may have to be undertaken again:

> A psychiatrist with retinitis pigmentosa was rendered blind as he was completing his residency training. He pointed out how long it had taken him to learn to negotiate his way to his office. Now that the building in which his practice was located was being sold, he was forced to move. This was a major hurdle for him, because it would require weeks of retraining to successfully learn the new route to his office (i.e., negotiating the curbs, street lamps, stairs and unexpected problems of urban traffic). As he said, "I usually have a weekend when I let myself get redepressed about all of this. I'm anticipating a lost weekend as soon as I know what's involved."

Thus, dealing with the never-ending demands of the environment requires a steady portion of the physically impaired person's daily energy. Within that, however, sudden environmental changes or transitions produce additional stress, demanding additional effort and energy.

**The "hidden" costs of community living.** Consider the following example:

> J.M., a 45-year-old psychiatric social worker, developed polio at 2 years of age and was rendered functionally quadriplegic. Although he completed several rehabilitation programs, very little mention was made of the fiscal realities of life in the community. Nonetheless, through dint of massively persistent personal effort, J.M. has built an effective private practice as a social worker for himself. However, in order to function, an enormous outlay of financially expensive support services is necessary. J.M. spends about $50,000 annually on needs related to his physical impairment. A special van with a life of no more than half a dozen years requires between $5,000 and $10,000 worth of special life accessories. He must spend $15,000 to $20,000 a year for drivers to both pick him up and deliver him. An electric wheel chair costs in the realm of $2,000 and also has a limited life. All this is in addition to ordinary and extraordinary medical expenses. He lives in continual anxiety about being so dependent on his driver-aides, many of whom have been unreliable in the past. In an interview with one of us, J.M. complained

ruefully that many medical professionals seem unaware of the barriers that exist in the community, not in the least of which are financial barriers, and the paradox is that as a man earning an independent living, he is unqualified for any financial assistance whatsoever.

## The Family, the Job, the Social Milieu

While many of the psychological burdens faced by former patients in the earlier phases of rehabilitation treatment are similar to current burdens faced by former patients now in the community, several are vividly different. Particular attention will be paid to issues of family functioning, the marketplace, and societal attitudes.

**The family.** Families face enormous burdens of renegotiating new roles, new boundaries, new equilibria, new sources of pleasure, new solutions to disappointments, and in some ways, new styles of relating to one another as the result of the profound change in the role of the newly physically impaired member. Families also have their own mourning to do and their own struggle to effect reality-mandated changes. Families must deal with resentments generated by their new role assignments. These assignments place restrictions on their freedom and demands on their time, and force them to learn about the bureaucracy of the service delivery system. They must learn, for instance, to negotiate with health care and finance agencies, each with its own boundaries, turf definitions, and idiosyncratic entrance qualifications.

When a family member is discharged from the rehabilitation setting, tremendous shifts in family routines occur. Although many activities designed to establish competence and familiarity with certain routinized processes have been adequately practiced in the rehabilitation setting, once the person is discharged, the family caregiver cannot simply call for help if he or she finds that an activity has begun to involve unexpected and unanticipated complications.

For example, sexual activities between spouses, once routinized and predictably pleasurable, can now be filled with anxiety and discomfort. The psychological pain of having a physical impairment can isolate spouses and lovers from sexually expressing their feelings. The result is a pervasive loneliness and despair. New ways of giving and receiving physical pleasure need to be learned, but risks need to be taken and time must be allowed for finding these new ways.

Listen to the words of a young couple who learned to overcome physical disability in their sexual relationship (Lenz and Chaves 1981):

Bob, a quadriplegic, broke his neck at age 16. He says this about his early experience: "My eunuch years also included a lot of martyrdom. I remember deciding that if I ever really fell in love with someone, I would end the relationship because I thought, being in a wheelchair, I could never really make anybody happy . . ."

His partner, Bernice, says this: "One of the advantages for me, of Bob not being physically able to do some things, is that he's gotten in the habit of asking for what he wants. It's great when he says, 'I'd really like to make love,' because I know what he wants . . ."

Bob responds: "Simply letting your partner know that you'd like to make love sure sounds easy now, but it was scary for a while. What if she said no? Some did. Then how would they feel about putting me to bed, undressing me, and dealing with my catheter and my spasms and on and on and on. . . . Before I broke my neck, orgasm *was* ejaculation. I took a long time to emotionally unlearn that, even after I intellectually knew the difference between the two. Now orgasm is more emotional than physical for me."

Bernice says: "Bob's great to cuddle with. His body is almost always really warm and I'm usually cool, so I love to wrap myself around him or scoot up behind him and sleep spoon style. Besides, I love feeling his skin against mine."

Bob ends this discussion by saying he knows he is a better lover now than he ever was before.

**Stereotyping and stigma.**    A stay in a rehabilitation facility tends to shelter the patient from the common experience of stigmatization or rejection (and postpone his or her exposure to this experience). Unhappily there are a large number of individuals who are either uneducated, unempathetic, fearful, or otherwise unable to deal with their feelings toward an individual with overt evidence of bodily damage. Stereotypes based on fear still abound, especially among those who do not have daily working or social contact with individuals who are physically different from themselves. Such people lack the ability to discern the unique humanness of the person behind the physical disability. Impairment by some is felt to be "contagious," and a person with such an impairment is often seen as inherently weak or morally inferior (Asch and Rousso 1985; Worthington 1977).

One vexing problem that some impaired individuals encounter when interacting with people in the able-bodied community has been called the "spread-phenomenon" (Goldman 1978)—that is, the perception by the able-bodied that individuals with a disability in one sphere are totally impaired in all areas. One person with a physical impairment described it thus: "When I am at a restaurant with an able-bodied woman, a waitress may turn to her and say, 'What will she have?'

(assuming I can't talk). Sometimes a stranger will walk by and pat me on the head and say 'It's good to see you out'" (Goldman 1978, p. 187). A blind person is often shouted at by others on a busy street corner, the implication being that one who cannot see, probably cannot hear either. After a few such wounding experiences, it is tempting for persons with physical impairment to withdraw from the wider world. Yet sometimes able-bodied persons manage their anxiety about the disabled in exactly the opposite manner, that is, through positive stereotypes associated with physical disability. The person with a disability can be thought to be saintly, courageous, and/or especially empathetic, or can be assumed to possess great psychological gifts (DeGuire 1990).

Social stereotyping is especially common in work situations when an individual with a disability is first introduced into an able-bodied group. This anxiety-induced stereotyping can lead to efforts designed to isolate, humiliate, scapegoat, or provoke, all of which can make it impossible for this individual to continue working. Occasionally the stereotyping will be silently supported, if not initiated, by a belief system on the part of management that physical impairment implies a mental impairment as well. Thus, persons so disabled cannot be hired or trusted to do any kind of work except the most menial or routinized.

An especially illustrative avenue to understanding social stereotyping is to consider the reaction of patients to physically impaired caregivers. B. Lawn (1989), a paraplegic physician who has specialized in psychiatry, describes a wide range of patient reactions to her condition. She understands them as the paradox inherent in the role of the disabled physician. To be disabled is to be seen as inferior, whereas to be a doctor is usually to be seen as powerful. Many of Lawn's patients had difficulty integrating these opposing concepts. Some of her patients assumed that because of her disability, she must be a poor doctor. Others assumed that because she was a doctor, her disability must be put on. It is not difficult to gather evidence to support the notion that social stigma about persons with physical impairment is alive and well in the community. The unpredictability of these encounters and reactions is an inevitable factor, making return to the community stressful. When individuals with impairments are asked about the greatest obstacle that they confront in their lives, the reply usually comes back as a single word: "Attitudes" (Hahn 1983).

**Architectural barriers.**    The idea of changing the environment to enable individuals with physical impairment to participate in society has been a long time in coming. For years, the public's unspoken attitude was that people with disabilities should be cared for somewhere out of view (i.e., kept in the closet). Even though progress has been made, much remains to be done. The Vocational Rehabilitation Act of 1973 provided the impetus to enforce an existing law to remove architectural barriers, but many regulations remain contradictory, if enforced at all. For example, while amendments to this law in 1976 mandated accessibility in airports, other federal regulations prohibited persons with certain impairments from traveling on planes without an attendant; and pilots are still permitted to refuse to carry patients with physical disabilities under certain circumstances (Hahn 1983). Not until 1982 did the Architectural and Transportation Barriers Compliance Board issue minimum guidelines for accessible design for federal buildings.

Ambivalence abounds in this field. In a major city in the United States where a member of our committee is on the faculty of a medical school, there are curb cuts for wheelchairs on all curbs surrounding this particular medical school. But only 2 miles away in the neighborhood that houses the site of a second medical school, there are virtually no curb cuts. Another example: The Americans With Disabilities Act of 1990 reinforces the decisions of the Architectural and Transportation Barriers Compliance Board to require adequate transportation on public conveyances for individuals who use wheelchairs. Nevertheless, the transportation authorities in virtually every American city of over 1 million resisted vehemently the expectation that buses would be modified or train platforms altered to make these forms of transportation accessible to persons in wheelchairs.

**Rehabilitation and work.**    Relatively few seriously disabled persons who return to the community are as fortunate as Mr. Hofsiss, the theater director, whose situation was discussed earlier in this chapter. Only one-third of physically disabled individuals in the United States return to work in the community. Those who do succeed in reentering the workplace are younger and have a strong prior work history. Unfortunately, the return to work may be a matter of years rather than weeks (Cogswell 1968). Despite the increasing utilization of vocational guidance and counseling programs, the results are modest. Why is the record of placement in this country so poor? Aside from the transportation and architectural barrier problems, there are several reasons for this.

Rehabilitation programs developed in the United States differ from their European counterparts in several crucial ways. In other countries, a person is initially certified for rehabilitative services based upon diagnosis and need; only if the rehabilitation proves unsuccessful is the individual then certified for some form of special income maintenance program. In the United States this process is reversed. Rehabilitation cannot be undertaken until a finding of physical disability is made and funding is guaranteed (Smith and Behart 1981). The definition of disability is linked to the standard of "an inability to engage in substantial, gainful activity," that is, means based rather than (medically) need based. This conundrum leads to a profusion of regulations that severely limit the nature and scope of rehabilitation services.

Even more troublesome is the assumption that the ability to work is determined principally by the individual's physical capability and is not the result of specific interaction between the individual and the workplace. Thus, too many rehabilitation programs are designed only to change the individual with a disability and not to match the individual to a modified workplace, that is, to alter the environment in which that person may be located. This narrow orientation fails to take adequate account of the wide-ranging talents that people with physical impairments possess. It also ignores technological advances and labor-saving devices that might make employment possible even for the severely disabled homebound or institutionalized individual (Hahn 1983). Although our country has made significant progress in this direction relative to 25 years ago, it still has a very long way to go.

As emergence of a philosophy of equal opportunity and nondiscrimination encourages optimal interaction, a portion of the economic problems of the disabled is slowly starting to change. The recent passage of the Americans With Disabilities Act of 1990 (PL 101-336) significantly changes the employment landscape by affecting all employers of 15 or more employees by the year 1994. This law requires that employers provide "reasonable accommodation" to the known physical limitations of an applicant unless the employer can demonstrate that such an accommodation would impose undue hardships on the business.

There are major disincentives that militate against individuals who are on income maintenance payments to abandon their benefits by seeking regular employment (Berkowitz 1981). Many people with such impairments are specially susceptible to catastrophic medical costs and therefore prefer to continue to accept meager social service disability insurance support rather than lose government health care protection provided by that support. In turn, unions are reluctant to take on people with physical impairment for fear of raising all their employees' medical insurance rates. Consequently, many people with physical disabilities have few opportunities for significantly increased income or upward future mobility in the marketplace (Feagin 1975).

The result of all this is that America spends approximately 10 dollars on dependent services for people with disabilities for every dollar it expends on programs to help them become independent (Bowe 1980). Hahn (1983) argues that the persistent residues of paternalism are a major cause for this tragically self-contradictory service policy.

## The Caregiver in the Community

Having sketched some of the difficulties the transition to community reintegration poses for individuals with physical impairments, this same landscape is now examined from the viewpoint of the caregiver.

The burdens for caregivers arise from the roles and functions they assume in assisting individuals with physical impairments in the struggle for community reintegration. Community caregivers soon become aware of the overall personal, social, and cultural worlds of those in their charge. Despite the particularities of professional role, most caregivers provide several broad categories of generic service:

1.  As educators, caregivers teach individuals with impairments and their families to anticipate barriers to community acceptance. Assistance in a variety of ways is offered in meeting the array of day-to-day problems of adjustment in the community.
2.  Caregivers provide encouragement and support through human involvement and through that particular form of empathic relating that involves standing alongside the patient and accepting the patient's experience and feelings. Above all, caregivers attempt to understand as much as possible about the daily rhythms and patterns of the lives of their patients. Caregivers attempt to detoxify the often immobilizing outrage felt by the person with a disability at the craziness of the barriers in the health care and service delivery systems.
3.  Caregivers often act like coaches or consultants, offering techniques and approaches whereby the physically impaired person can learn to exploit those systems constructively. In part, good community caregivers act as "hustlers" for persons with impairments and teach them how to hustle for themselves.
4.  As advocates, caregivers may become politically active in trying to achieve equality of opportunity for those persons with physical disabilities. At a more individual level, the goal is to help persons find the resources within themselves so that they may gain real control over their individual lives. The problem is that by taking leadership in these activities, caregivers may well fall into a subtle form of paternalism that actually impairs the individual from taking the more appropriate steps toward autonomy. Caregivers should be guided by the principle that ultimately they will have been so successful that they eventually disappear, that is, become redundant.

To what kinds of burdens then do all these activities subject community caregivers?

1. Anxiety is always present and is due in part to an identification with persons who must learn to operate alone or with a minimum of support. Community caregivers run all the risks of the isolated, lonely, seat-of-the-pants individual operating largely by himself or herself and making major decisions without benefit of an extensive team support system or backup hierarchy.

2. Community caregivers become the singular focus of all the psychological needs and demands of those they assist. This is decidedly different from the situation faced by hospital and institutional caregivers, in which the intensity of patient need can be split among the many different available individuals. In the community the single caregiver, whether social worker, psychologist, physical therapist, visiting nurse, minister, etc., may be the only caregiver that the disabled person sees for weeks on end. The emotional stress and the intensity of reactions described in Chapters 3–5 can be greater than when the caregiver works in an inpatient setting. Community caregivers are especially vulnerable to exhaustion, self-doubt, and disappointment, all of which they have to handle by themselves.

3. The caregiver in the community not only receives intense emotional demands but also faces a wide diversity and array of issues that the physically impaired person may present on any particular day. Many of these demands or needs transcend the boundaries of one's specialty. Persons living in the community expect the caregiver to be not only available and responsive but smart—that is, to have a huge data bank of tactical ideas and information on community resources. These kinds of expectations can leave any caregiver feeling threatened, if not helpless.

4. Former patients now living in the community can look on a community worker in an excessively idealized way in the beginning, as if this community-based helper can solve all their problems; fix everything; get them all the equipment they need that could not be gotten in the hospital; get them all the financial income support that could not be gotten while they were in the hospital; fix up their families so that they will not have any struggle to rebuild or reorganize relationships when they are living at home, etc. This "genie in the bottle" (see Chapters 2 and 5) relationship can happen in community settings as well. Caregivers are tempted to defend themselves from these pressures by limiting contacts with such persons.

What can community caregivers do about this? A few generalizations and some solutions are offered. On an individual basis, community workers may take special pride in the unique talents that they possess and that lead them to choose such work. Among the temperamental qualities needed are an ability to be comfortable operating relatively alone; a capacity to operate with trial-and-error empirical approaches; supreme confidence in the ability to find "some" kind of solution to most problems; and an ability to be excited by the challenges of the diversity of needs and desires in those they serve. Overall, community caregivers have to be comfortable being "generalists" and must have some kind of personal support system available to them to sustain them over time. Nevertheless they should not be afraid to ask for extra help when needed.

Emerging more recently as a way of improving service for individuals with complicated medical and social needs in the community is the concept of the *case manager*. Such a person assists the individual in "threading the maze" of the service delivery system. The case manager can streamline appointments while keeping long-term goals in focus. Those persons involved usually report positive experiences with case managers. The hallmarks of good case management include effective advocacy for the client, efficient communication with a variety of health care providers, and a knowledge of the likely routes to long-term success. Physicians rarely have the time or breadth of system-savvy to function in this intermediary role. Competent case management can serve the same role as a weekly case conference does on an inpatient service—that is, bringing all information and providers metaphorically "together" and keeping the methods and goals of community rehabilitation matched.

## Peer Group Support

Community caregivers are always on the lookout for potential resources for former patients who have now returned to the community. Social isolation, loneliness, and a feeling of worthlessness are constant threats to those persons with a physical disability. Our committee has had the most experience with groups as an important community resource. Described in this section are a number of group activities familiar to us.

For a person with a physical disability, groups are a vital caregiving modality in the community adaptation process, whether professionally led or self-help–oriented; whether diagnostically specific and restricted, or nonspecific; whether for persons with impairment only or for their families as well. Human beings are social creatures, and peer group activity for persons in the community is a naturally evolving foundation for successful community adjustment. Some individuals will, of course, become successfully adapted entirely by themselves with a minimum of help, but for the majority of individuals, that which replaces the array of team services and of structured social relationships in the hospital is not an analogous array of those professional structures and relationships in the community. What replaces the social, interpersonal, and group context functions of the hospital is the social network in the community. The group can be a vital part of that social network.

Groups serve as many functions as there are types of groups. Groups counteract the threat of social isolation, a major obstacle to community adjustment. It is all too easy to allow one's impairment to separate oneself from others or to hide in embarrassment and bitterness. Groups provide a bridge to other individuals (i.e., parents, other adults with disability) and make it possible for individuals to meet others who have traveled similar roads, experienced similar obstacles, felt similar anxieties, and solved similar problems. The realization that one is not alone is a potent source of psychological support. Such support may be a nonverbal expression: a sigh, a nod, a look that suggests, "I know what you mean," or "I know what you're going through." Such interactions help another feel connected and/or understood. Participants in groups often express the importance of sharing experience, of feeling supported, or of reaching out, as well as of the opportunity to get a variety of responses to pertinent issues. After a group formally stops, informal networks of former group members often continue to meet socially for months or years (Meyerson 1983).

## The Self-Help Group

Even in self-help groups, professional caregivers are often asked to play particular roles as teacher, guide, and, sometimes, consultant in order to assist persons in an ongoing adjustment to their impairment. One of us had the opportunity to meet with a group of 12 persons who were facing blindness. This group, which was initiated by a group of ophthalmologists for their patients, was assembled to assist individuals in adjusting to their condition. Vision of the individuals in this group varied from one man who was totally blind due to diabetic retinopathy, to several persons who were almost totally blind but could see some light, to several persons who had modest retinal damage but who knew that ahead of them lay the disparate fear of what they called "the great blackness." The first issue that confronted this group was an attempt to find an appropriate name. The underlying struggle was to name their group in as benign a way as possible, giving it a label such as "The Eyes Have It." In this first phase, the group avoided an open discussion of blindness per se. Initial sessions were used in discussing the practical difficulties of getting around in their homes so that they could cook and take out the garbage.

As the group members became more comfortable with each other and the consulting psychiatrist, they "tested" the consultant on his prior experience with others who had visual difficulties. They then felt free enough to begin to share their criticism and frustration with the doctors treating them. They wanted to know, for example, why doctors did not make it clear that the laser treatments were painful. This ventilation of anger on the physicians seemed to move the group closer to the despair they felt about the inevitability of their own visual loss. The consultant rephrased and clarified some of the underlying feelings that were being more openly expressed. This group continued to meet for one full year.

As time went on, the group seemed more and more to be composed of three types of individuals: one subgroup preached absolute active coping; a second used the group primarily to discuss their feelings of despair; and the third subgroup were seeking a way of accepting their impairments. The consultant helped to define, legitimize, and modulate these different themes over the course of the group experience. Underlying all the above issues was the coming of the "total darkness" for most of these group members. However, the one group member who was totally blind was able to convey to others his persistent sense of the joys of life itself.

Another type of self-help group with which our committee has had some experience is a group of former burn patients. Such a group was formed to ease the transition back into community life for the afflicted individuals. Because of cosmetic disfigurements associated with burn injuries, a major problem is withdrawal into a lonely and bitter isolation. Similar themes and a similar process occurred in the burn group as occurred in the blind group. Initially, when a sense of trust in the group was uncertain, some burn patients declared that only another burn survivor could be of any help. Issues quick to emerge were the patients' recognition of their common humanity as individuals, their need to resume normal lives, their recollections of the pain they experienced, and their responses to the reactions of the community to their disfigurement. Again, what the group was to call itself proved to be important. There was a good deal of feeling that they should not call themselves burn "victims" but burn survivors or former burn patients. The group developed cohesiveness quickly as they dealt with the care they received, how they felt about the doctors who cared for them, the acknowledgment of their disfigurement, and their return to society in an altered condition. Often the group expressed anger at the way society focused on appearance, and they expressed the wish to change the nature of society so that they could be better accepted. Again, as trust developed, more ambivalence toward the physicians who could not cure them emerged. Even so, some group members defended the care they had received and noted how helpful their caregivers had been.

One theme that was not anticipated in the burn survivor group proved to be very important: sexuality. The group members talked quite openly about how the loss of sensation of the skin or the change in their appearance had altered their sexual functioning. Group members shared new sexual strategies they used. The role of the professional in this setting was again to clarify pertinent issues and feelings and to legitimize options and choices so that more militant group members did not dictate decisions or opinions for the entire group. The consultant was, as before, a "guest" and not the group leader or convener. Running throughout the duration of this group was an undercurrent of anger at what had happened. The group seemed a relatively safe place to share this accumulated resentment.

## Psychotherapy Groups

A long-term group for patients with chronic medical illness was organized by one of our committee members as a formal psychotherapy experience (Stuber et al. 1988). The emphasis in this group was on the exploration of dynamic and interpersonal issues with leaders who are mental health professionals and who selected the membership through screening interviews. Members carried a variety of medical diagnoses and ranged in age from 29 to 63. Most of the illnesses were long-standing, with an average duration of 22 years. The group continued for 3 years and contained 14 members. Because of the diversity of group members, the expectations and needs of the group were also diverse. The group appeared to be used by the members in one of three ways:

1. *To foster psychological growth and development.* Several members used the group to discuss the psychological issues brought up by their disability or illness and "graduated" to new levels of comfort and competence.
2. *To provide ongoing support.* The largest segment of the members used the group for ongoing support and encouragement. They looked on the group as a "family" and would frequently refer to it as such.
3. *To provide atmosphere for further advocacy.* A few of the members eagerly joined the group, seeking others who felt similarly about important issues, but left after 1 year, feeling it did not offer what they were seeking. A key element appeared to be the way they defined themselves: as disabled rather than ill. Members defining themselves as disabled tended to be active in other organizations and working full time, and were impatient with the more dependent stance of other members (Stuber et al. 1988).

From a dynamic standpoint this group found relationship issues to be the most threatening, yet the most important issue broached during the 3 years of its existence. Members frequently sought advice and encouragement from one another about relationships, particularly with family members, such as parents or children. However, establishment and maintenance of intimate relationships appeared to be the most difficult topic. A common phenomenon was a brief discussion of one member's difficulty with intimacy, terminated by quick reassurance, or a rapid retreat into medication difficulties, or a discussion of the injustice of the social service system by other group members. Whenever the group was able to remain focused on the very real problems of isolation and alienation, the pain in the group became almost palpable, and it became impossible for the therapists to keep the group from fleeing the topic. With maturation of the group members, some interpretation of the defensive "fleeing" became possible.

## Recreational Groups

Groups can take more informal and recreational forms as well. In Minnesota the Courage Center began 50 years ago to provide recreational and camping experiences for those with physical impairments. Much of the Courage Center's initial public support came through these programs. As this organization has matured and grown, the more formal rehabilitation programs have come to the fore with goals tied to specific treatment modalities. Rehabilitation programs have threatened to overshadow the older recreational and camping programs that had proven so successful. The reason is that recreation is not considered "therapy" and is hard to justify for reimbursement. For instance, "respite care" is reimbursed, "play" is not. Although the benefits of recreational activities are hard to measure, staff members at the center are convinced that for many of their clientele with physical disabilities, the recreational programs provide more "results" (and an added incentive) than do the more formal rehabilitation or therapeutic activities (Voight 1989; R. Polland, Camping Director, Courage Center, Golden Valley, Minnesota, personal communication, 1990). The Courage Center believes that life should be fun, at least now and then, and the quality of recreation allowed the able-bodied should not be denied individuals with physical impairment.

In summary, groups of varying types (supportive, didactic, educational, recreational, therapeutic, self-help, etc.) are a powerful antidote to the social forces that tend to isolate individuals who have physical impairments or parents who have children with physical impairments. Not every group meets every person's needs, but, in general, groups have proven successful and their underlying concepts have been shown to be durable. It is important to help group members define their expectations and their needs as they enter the group experience. Caregivers may assist in not only leading such groups but facilitating their establishment and making appropriate referrals. Basic group experience appears to be a mixture of education/information, sharing of feelings and attitudes, and gaining insight about how one person is viewed by another.

## Conclusions

To live in the community implies that one is an important part *of* the community. Most people need an ongoing sense of belonging to something outside of themselves, whether it is a job, a cause, a group, or an intimate relationship. In this chapter we have emphasized the importance of caregiver relationships in assisting those persons with physical impairments to make the crucial transition from institution to the community. Caregivers may support, instruct, coordinate, advocate, and, when the time comes, step aside. Those with physical impairments require caregivers who can fill a need, provide a service, or otherwise resolve a problem without doing for persons with disability what these persons can do for themselves. In the face of these "special needs," is it surprising that community caregivers have special burdens?

A. Bartlett Giamatti (1989) stated it this way: "The paradox into which one gradually grows, through education and throughout one's life, is that independence is achieved through consenting to interdependence" (p. 14). As the individual with a physical impairment fights for his or her rightful place in community life and for an optimal degree of independence, that person's efforts must be supported and integrated by the community in which he or she lives, works, and loves. Every caregiver in the community is a social ambassador who expresses communal values and who often carries these burdens for all of us.

### The Doctor Rebuilds a Hand
(for Brad Crenshaw)

His hand was a puppet, more wood than flesh.
He had brought the forest back with him: bark, pitch,
the dull leaves and thick hardwood that gave way
to bone and severed nerves throughout his fingers.
There was no pain. He suffered instead the terror
of a man lost in the woods, the dull ache of companions
as they give up the search, wait, and return home.
What creeps in the timber and low brush
crept between his fingers, following the blood spoor.
As I removed splinters from the torn skin
I discovered the landscape of bodies,
the forest's skin and flesh. I felt
the dark pressure of my own blood stiffen within me
and against the red pulp I worked into a hand
using my own as the model. If I could abandon the vanity
of healing, I would enter the forest of wounds myself,
and be delivered, unafraid, from whatever I touched.

*Gary Young*

# 9

# Satisfactions

Given all the difficulties elaborated in the preceding chapters, one
might wonder why anyone chooses to take on the task of caregiver
to persons with physical impairments. In this chapter we will briefly
examine sources of caregiver satisfaction for those who have made this
journey.

The satisfactions caregivers can obtain in this work are legion. In
Chapter 6 it was noted that caregivers bring different skills, expectations,
and temperamental styles to their work. These styles closely parallel
subsequent satisfactions derived from the work. Some caregivers obtain
great fulfillment from intervening in acute lifesaving arenas such as
emergency rooms or surgical suites. Others find pleasure in the slower
process of helping people learn to feed themselves again. Some caregivers receive the greatest satisfaction when the disabled patient under
their care receives the first paycheck on a new job, and others rejoice
when one of their former patients is able to reach out and assist other
disabled individuals in a community setting. There is enormous room
for finding a sense of contentment in these endeavors, and each caregiver
may find it in different ways and in diverse places.

Caregiver satisfaction has a developmental component as well. That
is, as one matures in one's life the kind of satisfaction obtained changes,
although the work itself has not changed. This is one reason why
caregivers can find fulfillment in doing the same job for long periods of
time. Maturity often brings with it a readiness to find satisfaction in the
moments of patient-caregiver transactions. As one gains more experience, the "journey" becomes as important as the goals, or "destination."

We cannot attempt in this chapter to totally explain why caregivers
do this work. Satisfaction is not always predictable or even comprehen-
sible. There are those strange times when caregivers feel exhaustion or

emptiness when the situation would seem to call for a sense of pride, if not real joy. Then there are times of deep satisfaction in some momentary event that might seem to someone else mundane or trivial. Satisfaction can be one of those intangibles that surprise by their very unpredictability. However, there are some common sources of satisfaction, as will be explored in this chapter.

## The Chance to Make a Difference

When I went into nursing, I really wanted to help people. After a few years on the general floors, I felt like all I was doing was giving out aspirins. So I changed to physical medicine and rehab. What I like about this work is the chance to really make a difference. I can help someone go from nothing back to living. It's hard work, sure, and it doesn't always go as fast as we'd like, but I always know we've done something important.[1]

Making a difference is one of the most commonly cited reasons that people emphasize when they describe their work as caregivers. Individual personality styles will often determine which area is most satisfying to a given caregiver. People who want to see rapid progress and are more comfortable with brief, but intense interactions may find satisfaction in acute care settings (e.g., emergency rooms, surgical services). Others get gratification from teaching a patient to improve the function of a damaged hand in a rehabilitation setting. Still others find their fulfillment in the social activism of a community setting. Although the scope and pace vary with the setting, the common theme is the opportunity for the caregiver to use his or her own unique talents and energies to effect change. It is important for a caregiver to look around for the best, most satisfying niche, rather than to try to make do in a nonsatisfying area. The stresses of the work are sufficient to drive a caregiver out of the area altogether if the right match is not found fairly early (i.e., actually within a few months).

Most caregivers find themselves ready to move on to other areas of work after a few years. Rather than moving out of work with those who have physical impairments, caregivers may find it worthwhile to consider switching to a new area within the field. A move from direct service to administration (or vice versa), or a move from acute to long-term care, can allow the caregiver to apply experience in a new area while still feeling fresh. The satisfying sense of making a difference can also be enriched by partic-

---

[1] The remarks in quotation throughout this chapter are paraphrases of comments made to the committee members by clinicians in various settings.

ipation within a team or organization. In this way the caregiver's own voice is amplified and his or her own skills supplemented, and greater goals can be accomplished. An effectively functioning team can thus greatly increase the satisfaction of the individual caregiver.

Teaching also provides a way to make a difference that reaches beyond the individual, extending the skills and knowledge of one person by educating new caregivers. Watching students learn, grow, and begin to develop new techniques or ideas is a source of deep satisfaction. Teaching also provides a productive alternative for caregivers who find full-time clinical work too draining or who find themselves needing a change.

## Participation in the Patient's Struggle

> I had no idea what I was getting into when I agreed to teach post-amputation children to ski. But when I got to know some of these kids, and watched them take on challenges which would have overwhelmed me, I was hooked. They're amazing. I wouldn't trade those days for anything.

Sharing in the quiet, courageous everyday struggle of a person with an impairment can be inspirational. Caregivers discover how creative one can be in compensating for lost limbs, and how a determined person can learn to communicate despite a severe language deficit. Participating in these efforts with the patient is enormously satisfying. One can get past the moments of frustration, rage, or hopelessness as one rediscovers the human capacity to struggle against adversity. With the belief that problems can be addressed and either overcome, bypassed, or accepted, the caregiver and patient can assist each other in finding the strength and creativity needed to carry on. As the caregiver joins in the struggle against adversity, these interactions can restore the patient's faith in the fortitude and capacity of other people.

The major hazard in this source of satisfaction is overidentification (also see Chapter 5). Caregivers may get so involved in the struggle that they lose track of their own boundaries and find themselves either taking over for the person with a disability or becoming lost in the person's problems. To get close enough to join without merging is the objective and the joy. As mentioned earlier, a well-functioning team can help the caregiver maintain the continual awareness required to achieve just the right balance. Those caregivers who are able to accomplish this are very clear that it is well worth the effort.

This sense of comradeship in struggle can also be found in the inspiration and respect provided by colleagues. Many caregivers find that the high quality of their co-workers, and the satisfaction of learning and working together, are among the major gratifications they get from their efforts. While often overlooking their own talents, caregivers are likely to notice the courage and skills of their colleagues and feel privileged to work with those individuals who can challenge and inspire. Joining in a task with people whom one admires provides rewards not necessarily available in other settings.

## Feeling Special

People often ask me how I can do this work, and act like I'm some sort of saint. I'm certainly not! But I like the feeling that not just *anyone* could do what I do. I'm special.

Organizations like the Marines or the Green Berets have capitalized on the enthusiasm a group can generate if the members feel "special"—that is, chosen to do something not everyone could do. As discussed earlier, this "special" feeling can backfire if individuals come to believe themselves irreplaceable to the extent that they must make themselves available 24 hours a day, 7 days a week. However, when a group of people take pride in the work they do, knowing they do it well, then that group does better work. This is particularly true if the work requires special skills that are difficult to learn. A caregiver's sense of competence is enhanced by the awareness that few others could manage the task. The satisfaction of mastery of a difficult area is intensified by the work required to achieve that level of mastery. Well-functioning teams and wise administrators will make a point to recognize the competence and mastery of staff members.

Such satisfaction must be keyed to the *process* of the transaction rather than to concrete "results." Pleasure taken in one's ability to relate to people, to notice nuances, or to motivate provides much more stable gratification than counting upon specific progress. It is often the process of working with the physically impaired individual that provides the day-to-day rewards. Recovery or rapid progress obviously brings great pleasure but cannot always be counted upon to provide the ongoing satisfaction that a caregiver needs. This is particularly important for frontline caregivers. Direct contact with individuals who have physical impairments provides an opportunity for real satisfaction, but the satisfaction often comes only after some discouragement and frustration. This is to be anticipated and is a part of the daily vicissitudes of caring for a person who is struggling to change.

Being the "expert" in a particular area is very gratifying. Becoming known as an expert is relatively rapid if one works in an area no one else wants to study or attempt. The danger in this satisfaction is the temptation to really believe one knows it all. Elitism can destroy both the particular relationship with the patient and the relationships with the clinical care team. One then loses opportunities for further learning or growth.

## Meaning and Purpose

I talk with some of my friends, and their jobs seem so meaningless. They would probably laugh if I said this to them, but sometimes I feel like my work is a calling, a mission to fulfill. It gives my life meaning.

A sense of meaning or purpose provides extra energy within any work. An apocryphal story attributed to Henry James demonstrates this. Three men with shovels were digging in the same area in Manhattan. The first one appeared disgruntled and unhappy, and responded to the question "What are you doing?" with "I'm digging a ditch." The second one, who seemed somewhat more content, when asked the same question, answered, "I'm earning two dollars a day." The third man appeared clearly more enthusiastic than either of the others. He answered, "I'm building a cathedral."

Caring for the person with a physical impairment can certainly be seen in any of these three ways. For those who see a purpose in the work beyond just having a job, or a salary, the satisfaction is far greater. The meaning or purpose is highly individual and will vary within different settings and for different persons. Many persons will speak of their sense of participation in something larger than themselves and may experience this in religious, philosophical, or mystical terms. A caregiver may feel that his or her work is a moral act, a participation in the repair of the ecosystem, or a defiance of existential despair. The form does not matter as much as the significance. It is deeply fulfilling when one can find meaning in one's work. Providing assistance to people with physical impairments offers this opportunity.

Meaning can be found even within the most menial of tasks, when these tasks are seen within the context of the overall goal or purpose. As noted before, one of the ironies of work within a medical, rehabilitation, or long-term care setting is that the lowest status jobs involve the most direct contact with physically impaired individuals. If meaning can be found even within the daily grind of physical therapy, such work can be satisfying and fulfilling to the caregiver.

Holding on to the meaning can be difficult at times and requires the caregiver to be flexible. Acute care providers, for example, may find meaning in using technology to save a life or to prevent a permanent disability. However, such a definition of meaning leaves these caregivers vulnerable to incapacitating doubt if they find they have persisted in multiple invasive procedures past all hope of recovery. Meaning is more likely to be found as caregivers continually evaluate how to use technology in the best interests of the patient, and determine when to switch the goal from recovery to a more limited coping with the lost function. In some cases, the opportunity to learn something of value to future individuals can give meaning to a struggle that otherwise feels like a defeat. In a long-term setting, meaning can be found in ongoing day-to-day problem-solving work. Such a focus provides a sense of purpose that is sustaining not only for the immediate caregiver but for everyone involved.

## Being Needed

> I used to feel so helpless when they would ask me to come in at times of crisis. I finally realized that they really needed me there, and felt I was useful, even if I wasn't feeling like I was doing anything special. Once I understood that, then I could relax, and just do what I could, knowing it was as much or more than anyone else could do.

Being needed is one of the most powerful pulls any of us can feel. To feel essential to another person can be sustaining and create a sense of power and usefulness.

However, as discussed above, this is perhaps the most potentially dangerous source of satisfaction. The goal of working with a person with a disability is to help that person achieve optimal independence. Being needed is ultimately antithetical to this goal. As a parent gradually prepares a child to differentiate and separate, so must a caregiver allow and encourage patient autonomy. The temptation to infantilize is strong if one's major gratification comes from supporting someone who is dependent upon the caregiver. If, on the other hand, this satisfaction is balanced by the others just discussed, it can enrich, rather than erode, the interpersonal transaction.

The same is true for the caregiver in a teaching or administrative position. While it is flattering to have all decisions *need* one's input, it is exhausting and does not create good management or good learning. Students and employees must also be encouraged to develop and become more autonomous if the work is to progress.

## To Learn and Grow

When I started working in rehabilitation, I was all excited about helping these poor victims of disease or injury. It's embarrassing to think of how patronizing I must have been. What has really happened is that *I* have learned and grown in my interactions with these people. I'm not the same person I was, and I keep learning more everyday.

When a caregiver enters into the experience of a person with a physical impairment in a respectful manner, the interaction is enriching and enlarging for both individuals. Caregivers who allow themselves to see the patient as an individual with specific goals, strengths, and weaknesses, rather than as a victim, will feel admiration and determination, rather than pity and despair. This perspective does not come easily and necessitates self-examination and discovery of one's own biases, fears, and dreams. The reward for such internal work is personal growth and learning. Self-aware, reflective caregivers are productive and more able to work constructively with and for their patients. All of the sources of satisfaction are thus available to a caregiver who approaches the work in this way. Growth for both parties becomes the purpose and creates the chance for the caregiver to make a difference, participate in the struggle, and enjoy the specialness of his or her role.

## Conclusions

From the discussion above it can be concluded that it is not only quite possible but desirable to select one's work setting according to what is most satisfying for oneself. Persons who enjoy a nurturing role with a fairly dependent individual are best (for the good of all) in an acute care setting. On the other hand, those who find a deep, long-term relationship most satisfying will be most productive in a rehabilitation setting. Those who enjoy working with systems and making a difference on a community level will find satisfaction in a long-term care setting. It is extremely useful for caregivers to take the time and effort to discover such things about themselves. Rather than giving up on the entire field, many caregivers who are "burned out" could be resuscitated by a move to a different setting.

Providing care for people with physical impairments is not only necessary but extremely satisfying work. In this chapter we have discussed a number of possible sources of satisfaction. Potential hazards have been mentioned. The importance of knowing one's own strengths, needs, and sources of satisfaction cannot be overemphasized. Team and institutional support enables individual caregivers to achieve maximal effectiveness and satisfaction. Accompanying the patient on whatever part of the "journey back" that one is privileged to share thus contributes to a caregiver's wisdom and fulfillment.

# SECTION 3:
# EDUCATIONAL
# APPLICATIONS

## Doctors

They work with herbs
and penicillin.
They work with gentleness
and the scalpel.
They dig out the cancer,
close an incision
and say a prayer
to the poverty of the skin.
They are not Gods
though they would like to be;
they are only a human
trying to fix up a human.
Many humans die.
They like the tender,
palpitating berries
in November.
But all along the doctors remember:
First do no harm.
They would kiss it if it would heal.
It would not heal.
If the doctors cure
then the sun sees it.
If the doctors kill
then the earth hides it.
The doctors should fear arrogance
more than cardiac arrest.
If they are too proud,
and some are,
then they leave home on horseback
but God returns them on foot.

*Anne Sexton*

# 10

# Psychiatric Consultation
# in Rehabilitation

For most patients making their journey back from serious physical impairments, the services of a psychiatric consultant are not needed. But for some, consultation is crucial and a necessity. In this chapter we introduce the roles and functions of a mental health consultant in the rehabilitation setting. For purposes of efficiency, this person will be called the *psychiatric* consultant, recognizing that in some settings, that person may be a psychologist, nurse, or social worker by formal training. Nevertheless, many of the issues facing such consultants will be similar.

The consultant's role has a twin focus: patient-oriented consultative functions and staff-oriented liaison/educational functions. Suggestions will be offered that are equally applicable to both aspects of the work. The primary focus is the inpatient rehabilitation setting, with a secondary emphasis on the community setting. Specific staff educational functions will be left for the next chapter (on a model teaching program), and detailed tactical suggestions regarding the management of a psychiatric consultation will be omitted because such suggestions are available from standard psychiatric consultation texts (Pasnau 1975; Stotland and Garrick 1990). (For consultation specifically in mental retardation, see Group for the Advancement of Psychiatry 1979.)

When psychiatric consultants working in rehabilitation settings get a request to "please tell us what to do with this unmotivated and difficult patient," they know that their involvement is going to be complex, for it will encompass not only the behavior of a patient but the feelings and reactions of a number of staff as well. Thus, the consultant must attend to issues in the system as well as issues in the patient. Often such difficulties have been brewing over a considerable length of time, which also adds to their complexity. The "journey back" for some patients can be very difficult and may now involve old problems that predated the severe injury but are at this time resurfacing and causing everyone in the rehabilitation setting considerable pain. It is our feeling that psychiatric consultations in rehabilitation settings are both more multidimensional in their etiology and more far reaching in their consequences than in an acute care setting (Gunther 1977, 1979; Schwab 1982). While the focus here will be more on the specific ways the consultation-liaison psychiatrist functions as a participant/observer/educator in the system, we recognize that the foundation of this work is the accurate assessment and appropriate treatment of the involved patient's particular problems.

## The Origins of the Special Problems

In previous chapters the rehabilitation process with catastrophic illness was noted to generate expectable emotional crises in patients (i.e., "everyday psychopathology"). Such crises will be anticipated, recognized, and managed by the rehabilitation team. But what kinds of crises give rise to the need for *major or special psychological assistance* (i.e., a psychiatric consultation)? The essential guiding principle may be stated thus: Major assistance is in order when long-term efforts at the establishment of optimal rehabilitation goals and community stabilization of the patient are in serious danger of stalemating before achievement, or of being destroyed following achievement. The following rough classification of difficulties and their causes is useful in thinking about this principle:

1. **Preexisting major problems that are independent of current illness.** An example of preexisting problems would be an unrecognized affective disorder in a late adolescent or young adult, formerly managed by the "home remedy" use of significant amounts of alcohol during the day. Another example would be that of a depressed adolescent girl who is now spinal cord–injured as the result of her third and almost successful suicide attempt. Preexisting psychopathology is seldom alleviated by a catastrophic illness; on the contrary, it is usually worsened.
2. **Expectable problems of the rehabilitation patient as expressed by personality disorganization, regression, or intensely distressful feeling states greatly intensified by conflicts with caregivers.** Such patient/staff conflicts are usually cumulative and relentless. Examples might be the arousal of severe intractable emotional states such as rage, anger, hopelessness, helplessness, anxiety, fear, and disgust, and their overwhelming impact on patient/caregiver interaction. Or

patients may experience painfully immobilizing conflicts about the change in their bodies and the related task of evolving a new set of aims for their lives. Overall disorganization and regression to child-like states affect one's ability to reason, think, remember, and prob-lem-solve. This regression results in an inability to face the need to develop new vocational, social, interpersonal, or, at times, sexual role functions. It is crucial that these issues be attended to, lest the patient become sidetracked and fixated in a state of denial, disorga-nization, dependency, or some other kind of unmanageable chronic state. A frequently overlooked, but expectable consequence of failure to attend to these problems can be a patient's refusal to think about or participate in planning, let alone do the actual work of rehabili-tation. Instead, the patient waits, in the hospital or back in the community, either for miraculous restoration to normalcy or for someone else to do the planning, the thinking, and the work of the future.

3. **Paralyzing states of hopelessness due to desertion by crucial fig-ures in the patient's world, such as family and friends, or the absence of any meaningful support group.**

4. **Seriously conflicted working relationship issues between patient, staff, and/or family, or occasionally all three together.** These issues are seen in all medical settings (Meyer and Mendelson 1961; Schwab 1982). However, they tend to be more severe in settings that involve treatment of patients with catastrophic or major life-threatening illnesses. Certain patients can stir up in particular staff members intense feelings of anger. These feelings may be unrecognized and may involve prior problems that have nothing to do with the present dilemma (Gans 1983) but are complicating good care. Sometimes a staff member is humiliated by what seems an overwhelmingly hopeless situation and may react with a comment like, "Why should I bother working with such an ungrateful, uncooperative patient?" Caregivers may find it hard to recognize their underlying sense of helplessness in such a judgment.

5. **Breakdown of a once successful posthospital rehabilitation com-munity adjustment.** Once in the community, social supports are less visible and less structured when present, and the *overall demands on patients' own resources are much greater.* The causes of such stress here are protean (medical, psychosocial, vocational, economic, familial, etc.), but the final common pathway is some form of progressive multilevel psychosocial breakdown of the patient, who frequently becomes depressed and regressed and who may begin to drink excessively. For this pathway to be clarified and reversed, therapeu-tic intervention involves consultative skills as well as major integra-

tive efforts by the team and everyone else who can be usefully involved with the patient.

## The Many Roles of the Consultation-Liaison Psychiatrist in the Rehabilitation Setting

The professional responsibilities of the consultation-liaison psychiatrist working as participant/observer/educator in a rehabilitation setting with catastrophically injured patients and their caregivers are less certain, more complex, and more subject to situational variability than is the role of the same consultant in the acute care setting. First, the consultation-liaison psychiatrist will have to serve as consultant to the sick patient (in the context of all relevant social systems). He or she must be an expert diagnostician of the patient in all possible presentations. The consultant will, in addition, be competent in multiple therapeutic modalities: individual psychodynamic, milieu, interpersonal, psychopharmacological, and behavioral. This person may also have to function as consultant to the upper-echelon hospital administrators with respect to the psychological implications for both patient and staff of any new treatment program. In addition, the consultant usually serves as educator in a large variety of staff inservice training activities, both formal and informal.

Thus, the consultation-liaison psychiatrist typically plays several different roles. This can present a number of ethical dilemmas for which there are not simple answers. Toward whom is one's first allegiance— the patient, the family, the team, the administration? Our solution to the allegiance problem is to say that the consultant's primary responsibility is to the patient, but often *through* the team and the family, rather than directly. Troublesome examples are many, and only several will be listed here. First, the question of keeping secrets about some issue to which one of the staff members is not privy can be a real dilemma. Second, a patient begins to split staff into "good" and "bad" (as described in Chapter 5). Here the consultant helps the patient by attending to the system issue, in spite of the particular feelings the patient might have toward the consultant in that situation. Finally, a patient's need to hold on to some vestige of hope (although not realistic) is opposed by some of the staff who want the patient "to face the truth" and who want the patient's functional limitations described in objective terms. Here the consultant is in the middle of a system conflict and is charged with the responsibility of resolving it in a way that is both helpful to the patient and enlightening and useful to the staff. The reader will recognize that playing such a variety of roles that keep the patient's needs foremost requires not only insight but tact and diplomacy as well.

How does the consultation-liaison psychiatrist learn to do this? How does he or she learn which hat to wear at any one particular time and how to wear it? Many consultation-liaison psychiatrists who come to work in centers treating patients with catastrophic illnesses have some preparation for this type of work by virtue of their experience with such problems as loss, posttraumatic stress syndrome, and occasional contact with the victims of concentration camp traumas—all of which involve more than single-factor etiologies and single-modality treatment. There are several consultation-liaison postresidency fellowships in this country, and most medical school psychiatric residencies include some time allotted to consultation-liaison.

One of the essential features that any new consultation-liaison consultant quickly learns about this work is that people with catastrophic physical illnesses not only have suffered external losses (social role, etc.) but have lost part of themselves as well, both psyche and soma. Fully understanding the ramifications of this great loss is the central challenge for the new consultation-liaison consultant. From whatever backgrounds consultation-liaison consultants come, they soon recognize that work with people who have catastrophic injuries usually involves on-the-job training!

## Problems at the Interface

Whence do stalemate conflict issues arise that often require the attention of the psychiatric consultant in a rehabilitation setting? They may arise from within the staff system, from within the patient system (i.e., the family), from within the hospital system, or, at a distance, from the health care delivery system as a whole, particularly as represented by third-party payers (Mullins 1989). Usually the immediate situation requiring the consultant's attention is the interface problem; that is, the inability of the two principal systems—patient and staff—to communicate, relate, and work together constructively across a conflictual interface of different ideas, feelings, attitudes, and values (Gunther 1979). Consequently, the consultant's most urgent attention must be to the interface conflict, focusing his or her efforts in a manner that achieves the aim of restoration of the working relationship. The aim here is not to "cure" (either staff's empathic failures or a patient's psychopathology), but to restore broken communication and broken relatedness across the conflict-laden interface barrier.

What is the conceptual basis for such an attempt? In contrast to the most acute hospital work, rehabilitation hospital treatment is long-term (i.e., months instead of days or weeks). Therefore, relationships with rehabilitation staff must be thought of in such long-range terms. *The most important strategic aim is the restoration of feelings of worthiness and compe-tence to both patients and staff,* especially the sense of professional integrity of the staff. Typically, this integrity in the staff has been impaired by some degree of self-esteem injury resulting from the humiliating expe-riences of ignorance, disappointment, helplessness, or even despair. The net result is a basic failure in professional effectiveness (Gunther 1979). Assuaging such injury is the strategy that will lead to a restoration of a functional patient/staff relationship. *Restoration of the capacity for related-ness is the primary aim,* rather than the curing of anyone's underlying psychopathology or personal shortcomings.

The consultant's responsibility is to step aside and to look and listen differently, to see or hear what nobody else has seen or heard, or, if seen or heard, to elaborate the crucial significance of what has been seen or heard. Once a crucial piece of data not previously recognized has been found, it can then be used to repair basic relatedness. The central problem is most often failed understanding—either blocked, ignored, un-discovered, or disavowed. Without this addition of a crucial missing insight, all the systems theory or all the well-intentioned efforts at resto-ration of self-esteem will be to no avail. Some examples of unrecognized information elicited in our consultation experiences are the following:

1.  The spinal cord injury of one young patient was not the result of an accident, but instead indicated a disguised suicide attempt.
2.  A confused elderly woman patient was found to have a basic phys-iological problem of poor respiratory ventilation.
3.  A hysterically behaving adolescent who is extraordinarily frightened about "foreign" doctors was found to have been overprotected all her life.
4.  A brain-damaged adolescent girl who screams when certain male caregivers approach her was discovered to have been abused by her father when she was 6 years old.
5.  The patient who has trouble following instructions was found to have an IQ of barely 70.

Sometimes it is a previously unrecognized pattern or a combination of factors, as in the following:

1.  The patient must defeat our efforts to help her because no one, especially one who has been helpful, is permitted to become important to her.
2.  The nurse-therapist and her 60-year-old patient who suffered a stroke seem to be recreating the nurse's painful trauma with her own fatally ill mother.
3.  The patient is terribly agitated, but he is stir crazy from 11 months in hospitals without a home visit and fears his wife is abandoning him.

4.  The elderly man with a leg amputation has had a lifetime of relative failure, so why should he expect rehabilitation to be any different?

## Specific Tactics for Working With the Staff

The strategy of the consultation-liaison psychiatrist is to work with the staff through a series of everyday relationships with team and floor units. This approach builds mutual trust and respect. The consultant wins staff confidence by virtue of his or her willingness and ready availability to participate in daily struggles with patients. He or she also shares the staff's burdens and reactions by *working with them as a limited participant*, rather than by dictating to them. A combination of participation in everyday issues (i.e., "hanging around") and modestly offering suggestions for better management of staff's burdens, in addition to clearly expressed respect for the staff's level of competence, constitutes the best tactics for generating a reliable working relationship. Finally, the consultant must refrain from indulging in any condescending superiority (occasionally found among some mental health professionals). *Without this trust born out of a background of mutually positive relationships, all of the best advice, all of the best educational and inservice programs in the world, will ultimately fall on deaf ears.*

The consultation-liaison psychiatrist's relationships with the members of the frontline care team are crucial. There are no rigid formulas for gaining the respect of team members and for learning to work with them constructively. The best approach is that of exquisite courtesy and serious collegial respect built around the notion of "Do unto others as you would have others do unto you." There are a number of incorrect attitudes, such as turf guarding or exclusion of other professionals, that predictably lead to disaster.

## What Does the Consultation-Liaison Psychiatrist Have to Know?

The consultation-liaison psychiatrist has to know a great deal. With respect to the particular patient, one has to have an overall personal history, some current family and life situation assessments, and a current mental status examination. Next is the patient's medical history, including recent hospital experience as well as current expectations. The consultant has to know something of the other staff (the team), how they function and interact, how they relate to the patient, and what their basic attitudes are toward illness and rehabilitation. To what kinds of patients or illnesses are they particularly vulnerable? And one can only learn this by talking with key team individuals, utilizing the same serious, thoughtful care one does with patients. In addition, the consultation-liaison psychiatrist needs to understand the patient's concept of the disability and how this affects the patient's expectations and aspirations. How the illness will affect the patient's *future* is crucial, but in the hurly-burly of many rehabilitative settings the focus is more often on the *present*, and so the patient's future can go unexplored and not be made a part of the treatment plan.

There are other things the consultation-liaison psychiatrist has to know. Patients from different cultural backgrounds have different value systems and attitudes toward impairment, illness, health, recovery, exposure of the body, dependency, and the like. Different hospitals have different value systems that they impose on their staff, particularly with respect to what constitutes worthy behavior for staff and "cure" for the patients. For example, to what extent is the institution a prisoner of shallow performance statistics? How does the institution consider the psychosocial aspects of rehabilitation? What are their feelings about staff educational programs? In other words, the consultation-liaison psychiatrist must have a clear sense of what the value system is of the facility in which he or she works.

What else does the consultation-liaison psychiatrist have to know? Based upon the universal medical precept that rational therapy flows from some rational theory of pathology, the consultant has to know a great deal about the natural history of the particular disease in its developmental and dynamic consequences: how different pathological changes in anatomy affect life role capacities, self concept, body image, interpersonal relationships, etc. Knowing what kinds of issues arise with a 65-year-old stroke victim, or a 17-year-old victim of spinal cord damage from a gunshot wound, or an 8-year-old child with a malignancy, would certainly lead to vastly different treatment plans and specific psychosocial approaches to these three individuals. The details of how different disease groups affect anatomy, physiology, and basic capacity for life role activities will strongly determine the kind of issues that influence the patient's overall psychosocial adaptation to illness.

## Some Special Issues

### Pharmacology

The art of prescribing any significant medication to a person with a major disability is guided by the same rational principles that guide any prescribing of medication. There are, however, several simple warnings, perhaps better known from work with geriatric patients, that are equally applicable to a disabled population:

1.  Quantitatively, an adult with a physical disability is *not* just like any other healthy adult, but shrunken a bit in size and energy. Thus dosages should be prescribed accordingly.
2.  Qualitatively, every disability category produces its own unique metabolic/physiological/hormonal/enzyme alterations from the normal.
3.  The failure by caregivers to discontinue even questionably useful psychotropic drugs is the etiology of 20% of psychiatric consultation requests in a large teaching hospital's consultation-liaison service (P. Wright, personal communication to M. Gunther, 1988).

### Staff Referrals

What should the consultant do about referrals from staff members who ask for help about themselves? The sensible solution is to abide by the following principle: The staff member should tell the consultation-liaison psychiatrist enough so that the consultant can make an intelligent referral, but not so much that the staff member would feel humiliated or embarrassed by the psychiatrist with whom that person has to continue to work in the future. Consultation-liaison psychiatrists should not take into ongoing psychotherapy caregivers whom they are working with on a regular basis. It is important that consultants respect this role boundary.

### Psychotherapy

The question of direct patient referrals to the consultation-liaison psychiatrist for definitive primary psychiatric care must be handled judiciously and sensitively, as well as consistently with hospital and departmental policy. There are some situations in which the consultation-liaison psychiatrist may be the most appropriate person to treat a complex clinical situation, particularly those situations beyond the purview of other behavioral scientists from the team or beyond the purview of an "outside" behavioral scientist, who may never have treated someone with a catastrophic illness. Even under those circumstances, the consultation-liaison psychiatrist's activities should be limited to brief psychotherapy. Otherwise, the consultant risks compromising the centrality of his or her overall consultation-liaison responsibilities.

## Summary

Consultation-liaison work with patients who have suffered life-altering, appearance-altering impairments is both challenging and rewarding. The complex array of factors and the ways in which they interact; the diagnostic tasks of both patient and system; the uncovering of hidden issues that no one else recognizes; the task of designing an intervention strategy of appropriate effectiveness; doing one's work with little formal training or standard formulas—these are the challenges. And the rewards? The exciting opportunity to accompany and identify with a fellow human being's *struggle to overcome adversity* in the journey back is a reward that does not need much elaboration. In closing, a short poem sums up our feelings about this work:

> Life is short, the art long
> Opportunity fleeting
> Experience treacherous
> Judgement difficult—
> But the rewards are superb!

> *After Hippocrates/Goethe/Gunther*

# 11

# Three Proposals for Inservice Education

The material assembled in the previous chapters can serve as a reference source for a variety of inservice training programs in hospitals, rehabilitation centers, and clinics. Presented here are three possible course outlines for staff at various skill and experience levels. The focus of such inservice seminars is the psychosocial care of the patient. Much can be accomplished by having more experienced staff share the wisdom they have gained with less experienced, perhaps younger caregivers. For this to happen, the seminar leaders need to create an atmosphere of group trust and acceptance. The following materials can provide the initial content that could then lead to a fruitful discussion of patient management issues. Group leaders can easily include other written materials, videotapes, or demonstrations, and so forth, to amplify the territory covered in this chapter. An inservice pilot pretesting of these case vignettes among new staff at a well-known rehabilitation center in northeastern United States encouraged us to move in this direction.

The curriculum is divided into three parts, each corresponding to an experience or skill level that caregivers working with physically impaired patients commonly have. Curriculum A is for caregivers who have had less than 6 months experience in this field and who are learning about the special needs of such patients. It is directed primarily to staff on inpatient units. Curriculum B is for caregivers who have had more experiences with such patients and are dealing with the chronic stress of this kind of work. Curriculum C is for experienced senior staff and consultants who are now in a position as role models, teachers, or consultants for less experienced staff.

In all three curricula the primary teaching mode is the small group. In some sessions groups may get together for mini-lectures and in others, for informal discussions. The rationale for using small groups is to create a nonthreatening environment where caregivers can share their experiences of working with physically impaired patients. The groups work best if there are between five and seven members plus the leader. It is important that leaders be experienced caregivers who can ask stimulating questions in a nonjudgmental manner and focus the discussion on patient-related issues. Groups should attempt to reach a consensus on each management question before continuing to the next case.

Several key factors will determine the success or failure of this (or any other) inservice education curriculum. First, the administration of the program or institution needs to endorse and support this effort. The administrative leaders will need to be convinced that such an experience can improve caregiver satisfaction, reduce staff turnover or burnout, and improve interdisciplinary communication. In other words, such a course must yield some tangible improvement in the overall care system of the institution. If the administrative leaders feel that such programs only turn into "gripe sessions," they are not likely to be supportive. Administrative heads of departments or of the care facility will have to provide other patient care coverage while such courses are being conducted. This automatically incurs extra expense for the institution. So in administrative terms, it must be "worth it."

Second, such courses require strong leaders who will direct the discussions in fruitful ways. They not only must have experience and theoretical knowledge, but must know something about small group process. They must prevent the discussions from leaping into an exploration of someone's personal psychopathology or from allowing caregivers to displace and project their frustration onto the administration itself. The course should remain clinically focused and not be allowed to evolve into a political action group. This requires planning and the provision of clear expectations and structure.

Third, it is wise to build into any course an evaluation procedure. This approach provides feedback to the group leaders and some concrete evidence of what has actually been learned over time. No evaluation materials are included in this chapter. Such materials can easily be constructed by the leaders and tailored for their particular group.

Finally, the more interdisciplinary the support that such an effort has, the more successful it will be. If it becomes the province of only one department or group, it can easily be ignored or diminished in importance by others. Getting several key leaders to participate across disciplinary lines will automatically enhance the prestige of any such course.

# Curriculum A:
# An Introduction to the Physically
# Impaired Patient

## Goals

1. To normalize the reactions many caregivers have working with patients with physical impairments.
2. To understand the emotional stages that patients often experience following a major change in their capabilities.
3. To share the satisfactions and frustrations of this type of work.
4. To discuss the advantages and disadvantages of working on a multidisciplinary team.

## Readings From the Text

**Week 1:** Chapter 3: The Experience of Physical Impairment

**Week 2:** Chapter 4: Developmental Considerations

**Week 3:** Chapter 5: Caregiver Reactions

**Week 4:** Chapter 6: Coping Strategies

**Week 5:** Chapter 7: Therapeutic Transactions

**Week 6:** Chapter 9: Satisfactions
Chapter 12: Conclusions

## Format

There is a brief time requirement of approximately 6 1-hour sessions in interdisciplinary small groups. The focus is on discussion of case vignettes. The course can start with an introductory mini-lecture in which an overview of the course is given, including an explanation of the goals and group activity involved in the learning process. Later in the course is included a large group lecture/discussion session on the reactions patients often experience following a significant physical loss, emphasizing ways to understand the stages commonly observed in patients going through the rehabilitation journey. (Some of the vignettes are covered in the text and some are not.)

## Case Vignettes

1. You are working with a 10-year-old girl who has recently undergone an amputation of her leg at the hip because of a malignancy. She is vigorously fighting any and all attempts to introduce a prosthesis. She will not discuss anything that has to do with her rehabilitation.

   a. What are some possible hypotheses for this girl's behavior?
   b. What could you say or do to help her?

2. You have just returned home from work feeling tired, and a close friend asks you, "How do you do it? I could never stand that kind of work!"

   a. Have you had friends make this kind of comment?
   b. How do you respond?

3. A co-worker walks into the nursing station and says, "I really hate the new patient; what do you think of him?"

   a. Should caregivers ever hate their patients?
   b. If they do, should they admit it to other caregivers?

4. You walk into the patient lounge and overhear another caregiver speaking to a 30-year-old woman who has just been transferred from the acute care hospital to your rehabilitation facility. "You may not be able to walk now, but if you do these exercises every day, you'll be out in the 10K by next spring." You know that the woman has had an injury that makes it extremely unlikely that she will ever run again.

   a. What would you say to the other caregiver?
   b. What would you say to the 30-year-old woman?

5. A caregiver had worked for 10 years with a quadriplegic 65-year-old male. They had developed a close attachment. After the patient suffered a severe stroke, the caregiver felt depressed and bitter. She questioned whether she should continue in her present job.

   a. Is it wise to get so attached to your patients that you grieve their misfortunes?
   b. What could this caregiver have done to deal with her feelings?

6. "When I started working with physically disabled people, I was all excited about helping these poor victims of disease or injury. It's embarrassing to think of how patronizing I must have been. What

has really happened is that I have learned and grown in my interactions with these people. I'm not the same person I was, and I keep learning more everyday."

   a. What problems arise from viewing impaired disabled people as victims?

   b. Do you think that working with impaired people changes the way you view yourself? If so, how?

7. A 45-year-old mother of four is making no progress in her rehabilitation program for her chronic back pain. A caregiver says, "You're being a bad parent by not wanting to get on with the rehabilitation program. Think of what you owe your family."

   a. What predominant feeling did the caregiver attempt to elicit with this response?

   b. What other ways could this caregiver have dealt with his or her frustration?

8. A 10-month-old infant with a tracheal-esophageal fistula has been kept in the hospital since birth because of the necessity of tracheal intubation. Over this time the infant's caregivers have grown very attached to this child and occasionally bring the child gifts on special days. However, they also find themselves more critical of the child's mother and find it hard to be around her. This reached a crisis when one of the nurses asked for a psychiatric consultation because of the mother's "neglect."

   a. What predominant feelings in the caregivers are generating this conflict with the child's mother?

   b. Have you noted such feelings in yourself when you interact with members of a physically impaired child's family?

   c. Are such feelings expectable?

   d. What are some other ways the caregivers of this child could have dealt with their feelings toward the mother?

9. A 35-year-old divorced basketball coach, now in his 60th day of rehabilitation, suffered a spinal cord injury at T6. He has no sensation in the lower extremities and has concerns about his sexual function. Although he refuses to attend the sexual education group on the ward, he requests a sexually oriented touch from one of your colleagues to see "if it's all dead."

   a. What feeling in staff might be expressed in a team meeting about this behavior?

b. What variety of approaches could you think of to more appropriately respond to this request?

c. Could the staff role-play several of these responses during a team meeting?

10. You have worked intensively for months helping a teenage boy who had a moderate head injury. You have found his rapid progress exciting and gratifying. When the team thinks the patient is ready to start to focus on his transition back home, you have a deep sense that he is not ready yet. When you think about it again you realize that despite the joy of seeing him becoming more independent, it makes you sad to realize that each advance means he will be leaving soon.

a. Are there parallels between working with rehabilitation patients and being a parent?

b. Everyone wants to be needed. How can this universal desire be both an asset and a liability in working with physically disabled people?

# Curriculum B:
## Caring for Patients With Physical Impairments: A Psychosocial Perspective

## Goals

1. To normalize the stress involved in working with physically impaired patients.
2. To learn how to use subjective reactions to patients therapeutically.
3. To discuss how to work with patients who are hateful, angry, demanding, noncompliant, or depressed.
4. To recognize and learn to deal with patients who "split" caregivers.
5. To discuss theoretical models that can be used to understand the reactions of patients and staff to physical disability.
6. To share ways of dealing with the dilemma of distance versus identification with patient.
7. To identify useful coping strategies.
8. To share personal satisfactions (and frustrations) of working with physically impaired patients.

## Readings From the Text

**Week 1:**  Chapter 1:  Introduction: A Rationale

**Week 2:**  Chapter 2:  Conceptual Foundations

**Week 3:**  Chapter 3:  The Experience of Physical Impairment

**Week 4:**  Chapter 4:  Developmental Considerations

**Week 5:**  Chapter 5:  Caregiver Reactions

**Week 6:**  Chapter 6:  Coping Strategies

**Week 7:**  Chapter 7:  Therapeutic Transactions

**Week 8:**  Chapter 9:  Satisfactions

**Week 9:**  Chapter 8:  Community Living: The Final Destination
              (first section)

**Week 10:** Chapter 8:  Community Living: The Final Destination
              (second section)

**Week 11:** Chapter 12: Conclusions

**Week 12:** Course Evaluation and Wrap-Up

## Format

This curriculum covers the basic reading material as in Curriculum A, but also includes the material on community living (Chapter 8). More time is allowed for an in-depth discussion of the material covered. There are approximately 12 1-hour sessions. Large group discussion of cases take place and can be intra- or interdisciplinary. After a brief overview and discussion of goals, groups can begin on the cases during the first session. Intermixed with group sessions can be large group lecture/discussion sessions. Possible topics are as follows:

1. How can we understand the patients' psychological reactions to their disability?
2. When is it appropriate to get an outside consultation?
3. How can one avoid getting burned out?
4. How can the effectiveness of an interdisciplinary team be maximized?
5. Are there other topics of specific interest at one's institution that can also be discussed?

**Case Vignettes** (Some of these appear in the text and some are new.)

1. On a rehabilitation ward an acutely agitated 19-year-old adolescent paraplegic male, left paralyzed by a motorcycle accident 2 months ago, has a previous history of antisocial behavior. Following an argument with his girlfriend he holds a glass of water and threatens to throw it at one of the caregivers.

   a. Have you been in a similar situation?
   b. What feelings does this behavior elicit in you?
   c. What are several ways this situation could be handled?
   d. What might happen that could worsen such a crisis?

2. **Part I:** A 22-year-old woman was several weeks into her rehabilitation for a severe injury that rendered her right leg nonfunctional. She showed a persistent wish to be cooperative with her caregivers, never complaining, and always presented them with a cheerful smile. Yet, there was something in her demeanor that left her caregivers unsettled and unhappy.

   a. Have you been in similar situations where a patient's "cheerfulness" made you uneasy?
   b. Can you think of reasons why some patients behave this way?

   **Part II:** At a team meeting one of the staff mentioned that the patient's smile seemed brave but "fake," and she found herself as a caregiver irritated by the patient's "artificial" cheerfulness and attempts to act as if nothing very serious was wrong. Other caregivers concurred, stating they often felt exhausted after caring for her. Further team discussion led to the notion that this young woman might be rather depressed underneath her "brave front" and that the team needed to keep this issue in mind as they cared for her.

   a. Would it be appropriate to request a psychiatric consultation?
   b. Can you think of ways to give the patient permission to feel her sadness without embarrassing her?

   **Part III:** Several days later, one of her caregivers noted that this woman was getting irritated that her brace would not lock into place correctly. The caregiver said lightly, "Whew! I'm glad to see you can get angry once in a while. I was wondering where all those feelings were." The patient looked startled, then broke down in tears as she confessed how much she hated the whole lousy business of being in the hospital.

    a. Do you agree with what the caregiver said?

    b. What other responses might have been helpful in interacting with a patient like this?

3. A 35-year-old man who has 40% body burns is on your unit. You are responsible for changing his dressings daily, which he finds extremely painful and distressing. He begins to refer to you as "the ogre," but he likes the other caregivers.

    a. No one else has volunteered to help with the dressing changes. You do not like being the bad guy. Should you say anything to your fellow caregivers, your supervisor? Should you do nothing?

    b. What feelings does this patient elicit in you?

4. An 18-year-old girl has been on the rehabilitation service for 3 weeks. Today, in team meeting half the team want her to be discharged because she is so angry that some of the staff feel she cannot gain anything from being on the service. You and other team members agree that she can be outspoken but that her family is so disturbed, that it is no wonder she is angry. You think she needs to stay, perhaps even longer than usual, because of the lack of support her family can provide.

    a. What would you say to the team members who want to discharge this girl?

    b. If it is unusual for the team to be divided like this, what do you think is going on?

    c. How can this situation be resolved in the best interests of the patient and the team?

5. **Part I:** A 5-year-old child was hospitalized for severe burns with accompanying facial disfigurement. The parents noted a mechanical and impersonal aspect to the care the child was receiving and in some alarm complained to the head nurse. The bedside caregivers in turn complained that the child was so negative and irritable that appropriate responses were nearly impossible.

    a. As the patient's primary caregiver, what would you say to the parents? To the other caregivers? How could this case be discussed in a team meeting?

**Part II:** The parents bring in pictures of how this child looked before the fire. They also teach the caregivers about their daughter's interests in drawing and music.

    a. What other ways can caregivers and family members work together?

    b. How can caregivers keep the channels of communication open with parents and family?

6. A 25-year-old male patient with multiple injuries resulting from a severe car accident is confined to a body cast and has been in the hospital for 2 months. The staff know his wife has recently separated from him. They also note that he begins taking "liberties" in his interactions during bathing and routine care—that is, by slapping nurses on the buttocks as they walk past his bed.

    a. What are the main issues in the management of this patient?

    b. Does trying to put yourself in his shoes "lead you anywhere" in finding an appropriate response? Is using humor acceptable here?

    c. Would requesting a psychiatric consultation be warranted?

    d. How could a team meeting be used to solve this problem? Is the issue more than one of restraining his behavior?

7. A 35-year-old lawyer is attacked by robbers and left paraplegic. He is angry, angry with everybody. Much of his anger springs from the powerlessness this previously very powerful man is experiencing. Caregivers who try to soothe him or do things for him quickly learn that he is neither appreciative nor cooperative.

    a. You notice that you spend less time in this patient's room than with other patients with similar injuries. What might be the reasons for this?

    b. What interventions might help this patient and make it easier for you to care for him?

    c. How can the team be used to support you as the caregiver in this situation?

8. A fellow caregiver has been working on the spinal cord–injury floor for 3 years. No patient on the floor can be admitted without her being there. She is essential and everyone knows it. You are shocked when after a difficult night she comes up to you and says, "I'm so exhausted I think I'm cracking up. I can't take it anymore!"

    a. Do you know veteran caregivers who are indispensable like this?

    b. What is happening to her?

    c. What feelings does this elicit in you?

    d. What ways do you have of dealing with the pain and frustration of your work?

    e. How much of this do you share with your spouse, loved one, etc.?

9. A 12-year-old boy went swimming in an old quarry where his parents had told him never to swim, hit his head on a rock, and sustained a thoracic spinal injury resulting in loss of function of his legs. His parents do not seem to want to cooperate with the hospital staff, and, finally, one day the father asks you, "Why aren't you curing our wonderful son?"

   a. What feelings are elicited in caregivers when patients and/or their families use denial in coping with a serious injury?
   b. How important is it to "break down" this denial? What might be some reasons why this may not be advisable?
   c. What solutions might an interdisciplinary team generate in the face of this dilemma?

10. A 22-year-old male patient with a congenital bone disease is refusing to cooperate with any of the staff following a reconstructive leg operation, making most of the staff angry at him. Finally he tells a caregiver that no one here likes him so he is going to leave immediately.

    a. Because he is not a minor, should he be allowed to leave against medical advice?
    b. What feelings might lie underneath this patient's anger?
    c. Can you think of several empathic responses you might make in this situation?

11. "When I went into nursing, I really wanted to help people. After a few years in acute care nursing, I felt like all I was doing was giving out aspirins. So I changed to physical medicine and rehabilitation."

    a. Is this a common reaction?
    b. What kinds of caregivers prefer physical rehabilitation?
    c. What kinds of caregivers prefer acute care?

12. "No caregiver should solve a problem or do something for a patient that the patient is capable of doing."

    a. Are there exceptions to this rule?
    b. What are the dangers of always sticking to rules?

13. A 4-year-old girl who suffered a pelvic fracture began to suck her thumb, which she had not done for years, and began to wet her bed at night. Her parents were upset with the hospital staff for letting her act like a baby.

    a. What is happening to this patient? Is this a common response to hospitalization?
    b. What feelings lie *behind* the parents' being upset?
    c. How can you respond to these less obvious feelings?

14. A 91-year-old patient, who reminds you of your grandfather, often becomes confused at night and begs you not to attack him or take all his money every time you come into his room. When you try to reassure him he starts screaming for someone to save him.

    a. Why are elderly patients subject to such behavior?
    b. What are some things you can do to prevent the recurrence of these episodes?
    c. Would a psychiatric consultation be useful in such situations?
    d. What could be done at team meetings to deal with particular feelings generated by this patient?

# Curriculum C:
# Leading the Way in the Psychosocial Care of People With Physical Impairment

## Goals

1. To train leaders for Curricula A and B.
2. To share the stresses of being a role model/mentor for less experienced staff members.
3. To adapt these materials for the particular needs of the staff.
4. To learn advanced psychological models for understanding patient and staff reactions.
5. To learn effective use of the psychiatric consultant.

## Readings From the Text

All of the text should be read.

## Format

There is a moderate time commitment, approximately 8 1-hour sessions, with additional time needed if the group is planning to lead Curriculum A or B for their staffs. The group is small and usually interdisciplinary, but can be intradisciplinary if there are enough staff who would benefit from the course. Curriculum C may be the first one implemented at an institution as a springboard for generating a group of teachers for Curricula A and B. Curriculum C can be used with a wide range of professionals, including psychiatric residents and medical rehabilitation residents. Individuals who have not had significant experience working with patients with physical impairments should especially note Chapters 3 and 4. Cases in Curricula A and B can also be reviewed. Possible lecture topics are as follows:

1. Common dilemmas in consultation.
2. Transference and countertransference reactions in rehabilitation medicine.
3. How to improve one's leadership skills.
4. How to help a staff member who is having problems in the psychosocial sphere of patient care.

## Case Vignettes

1. A 25-year-old single female interior decorator suffered 20% burns over both lower extremities that require daily dressing changes. She insists that only you know how to change the dressings and is very upset when others attempt this. She praises your skill to her other caregivers and makes hostile wisecracks about them with you.

   a. What dangers does this situation hold for both you and your patient?
   b. What psychological processes are occurring here?
   c. What are some ways you can think of to handle this experience?

2. You are a consultant for a chronic pain team. A 40-year-old male caregiver on the team pulls you aside after one of the team meetings and says he is having troubles with his wife and wants to know if he can meet with you to get some advice on what to do.

   a. What do you say to him?
   b. He later asks if he can come to you for psychotherapy. What would your response be?

3. A 48-year-old widowed female homemaker with a complicated past history of chronic renal failure superimposed on severe coronary artery disease enters the hospital again for the third time in the past 6 months. She also has bouts of depression with recurrent suicidal

ideation and insomnia. The management question of sending her home versus sending her to a nursing home arises.

   a. What factors should be considered in making this decision?

   b. What contributions can her daily caregivers make in arriving at this decision?

   c. How could a psychiatric consultation be integrated with other information in such a situation?

4. You are consulting in a military hospital, watching a singular inter-action between a severely facially burned corporal and his nurse. The nurse, with a touch of sarcastic humor, refers to this man as "dog face." You notice a good deal of respect and closeness between the two in subsequent conversation.

   a. What kind of response is this nurse making?

   b. Does empathy always mean being nice to patients?

   c. Can you contrast empathy with pity? sympathy? fusion? Where does "I can relate to that" fit in?

5. You have been working intensely with a 48-year-old male patient (former truck driver) who sustained a serious head injury 4 months ago. He has bouts of intense anger when he cannot accomplish something and has recently threatened you in one of these outbursts. You surmise that he is angry because you push him harder to achieve his functional potential while other staff are more afraid of him and back off. A supervisor suggests you transfer to a different unit so you will be safe.

   a. What feelings arise in you as a caregiver as a result of this suggestion?

   b. What role might a consultant play in helping to resolve this dilemma?

   c. What other ways might the supervisor handle such situations?

6. **Part 1:** The medical rehabilitation resident angrily demands to know why the physical therapist has been unable to carry out the ordered treatment, and does not accept the notion that "the patient was unwilling."

**Part 2:** The team confronts the social worker with a demand that he or she get the particularly anxious and intrusive mother of a patient to have more appropriate and productive interactions with the staff.

**Part 3:** The team presents the psychiatrist with the demand that he or she motivate or discipline the disorganized patient into "behaving properly" (i.e., compliantly).

   a. What do these situations have in common?

   b. Can a patient's care be compromised in these situations? Have you seen an example of this?

   c. As a consultant or supervisor, what can be done to resolve these situations?

7.  A nursing student reports to her supervisor that a patient with whom she has been working is extremely angry at the staff and might elope from the hospital. When this is discussed in the next team meeting, no one else on the team has felt that this patient is angry. The student argues that she has spent a lot of time speaking with the patient, but the senior nurse who has worked with this patient does not seem worried. You are the team leader.

   a. Who is likely to have the best handle on this patient?

   b. How would you proceed in the team meeting?

   c. What plan could you elicit to resolve this difference of opinion?

8.  A 48-year-old professional country/pop musician with a 15-year history of multiple sclerosis comes to a rehabilitation center for brief periods of steroid therapy. His community rehabilitation worker feels he could do gainful work, albeit not as a musician. The patient's wife, who works full time herself, feels he is fine at home and does not want him on an out-of-home placement. The consultant is called to resolve this staff/family dispute.

   a. How do you think a consultant might proceed?

   b. How would you assess the patient's social networks?

   c. Would a home visit be useful?

9.  An 85-year-old woman with Alzheimer's disease and a fractured hip is on the rehabilitation service, and the team comes to the decision that it will be impossible for her to return to her independent living situation. The family disagrees strongly and says that the hospital is just giving up and should keep trying until their mother can return home. They threaten to sue the hospital if she is sent to a nursing home. A consultant is called in to help resolve this dilemma.

   a. Could this deadlock between the hospital staff and the family have been avoided? If so, how?

b. What underlying defenses might the family have used in reaching this conclusion about disposition?

c. The oldest son of the patient travels 1,000 miles to come to a family meeting and tells the staff adamantly, "If you really cared about my mother you would never send her to a nursing home." His sister tells him, "I don't see you volunteering to take her home with you! You haven't visited her for years!" How can you help this family?

d. Can you outline an operational plan of information gathering and conflict resolution?

**Our Credo**

We believe caregivers are chosen—
rather than choose—this work,
Because they can tolerate
suffering,
anger, neediness, and despair
And find enough
      meaning,
      hope, and
      satisfaction
To continue caring,
at least for a while.

Our mission is to increase both
tolerance and hope,
Without denying the reality
of the suffering involved.

This book is dedicated to that task.

*Margaret L. Stuber, M.D.*

# 12

# Conclusions

W hy write such a report? This question returned to preoccupy us as our committee completed this work. The final chapter provides us an opportunity to restate the core concepts and assumptions used in constructing this monograph. Part of the rationale comes from our organization, the Group for the Advancement of Psychiatry (GAP), itself. All GAP committees are enjoined to reevaluate old ideas and explore new avenues for the promotion of mental health in our society. Our committee felt that significant advances in both theory and practice regarding the effects of bodily impairment on psychosocial functioning had occurred in a number of disciplines, and that these ought to be integrated in a way that is of use to professionals who might not have extensive training in psychiatry. Previous works had often omitted dealing with issues particularly germane to general caregivers themselves. Our focus has been an attempt to correct this omission.

To provide an avenue for this reaffirmation of basic principles, a final vignette is provided.

Ms. H. was 20 years old and at the Coconut Grove nightclub with a date (in 1942) when she was terribly burned in that infamous fire. One of our committee interviewed her at the age of 62. In her interview, she could vividly recall the explosive outburst of flames and the ensuing confused panic of the trapped crowd. She was knocked down repeatedly as she fought her way toward the exit, aware that her feet and legs were on fire. Ms. H. described feeling unafraid at the time, being preoccupied with her father and anticipating his sorrow. She last remembered falling to the floor of the nightclub, prepared to die. She was taken to the Massachusetts General Hospital with second- and third-degree burns of all extremities, head, and chest. After a 5-month hospitalization and four surgical grafting procedures, she was discharged with extensive scarring of the face and chest, loss of the fingers of her right hand, and loss of portions of her scalp. Her boyfriend died of burn injuries.

When she was asked what she found helpful in coping with her burn injuries, Ms. H. unhesitatingly responded, "My nurse and my surgeon." She credited her nurse with "saving my sanity . . . she treated me as if nothing was wrong with me; she was rough and humorous, but mostly she was always there for me." Her surgeon, according to Ms. H., "made all the pain endurable because he cared so much." She recalled him holding her bandaged hand, explaining the situation to her in detail, and "making me feel protected." While the interns removed the bandages he would stand at the head of her bed and instruct her to cry out and scream. "Of course, I couldn't," Ms. H. remembered, "but it made me feel brave, especially when he said, 'I know what you're going through.'" Later, Ms. H. would name her first son after this surgeon.

Ms. H. was not aware of the extent of her burn injuries until after the fire. Her nurse sat her up, naked, in front of a mirror. "I never thought I looked so bad until I faced the public." The reality of the loss hit her as she observed people's reactions: "My former dates disappeared, children were terrified of me, one friend fainted when she saw me, and everybody stared. I just smiled, but I felt like killing myself."

Now, at age 62, Ms. H. reflects: "It never leaves you. You try and forget and stay busy, but it never leaves you." She acknowledges that she has been viewed as a success: "Everybody says I am so brave and well-adjusted, but inside I've never accepted the physical scars. Time hasn't helped. I find myself reliving the fire and the hospitalization all the time when I'm alone. I still miss my fingers and hair terribly."

This journey back from life-threatening injury and residual disfigurement contains within it most of the issues that have been emphasized in this report. They are reiterated here:

1. **Caregiving activities transcend the particularities of time and circumstance.** Even though the fire and the injury occurred 40 years ago, Ms. H.'s account has an immediacy and vividness that makes one feel this could have occurred yesterday! Although the distress of her physical disfigurement continues to live on over time—one can never delegate injuries completely to the past—so too does the power of the caregiving relationships established long ago, seeming to have an equal life of their own. Ms. H.'s memories keep both the impact of her near-death injury alive and the care she received to deal with the trauma. It seems to the reader as if the experience of her past care provided a kind of ongoing nourishment, a reservoir of emotional courage in order to face the anguish of her subsequent

impairment. What caregivers do takes its place alongside all other life experiences, but rarely is it routine or insignificant. In the mind and memory of the patient, care often transcends its particular circumstance. Patients can retrospectively uphold such interactions with caregivers as an important source of strength and encouragement. Such caregiving activities enshrine themselves in the patient's mind, as was true for Ms. H.

2. **Caregiving rests on a real human relationship.** Ms. H. credited her nurse with being "always there for me," and her surgeon for "making me feel protected." It might seem trite to emphasize that all caregiving rests on a fundamental relationship, but in contrast to acute care activities, which often occur only over hours or days, caregiving of the kind discussed here occurs over weeks, months, and even years. Sustained contact with patients as they heal provides opportunities for these relationships to develop. As Ms. H. shows so well, these transactions take on important psychological dimensions for the recovering patient with a physical impairment. A sense of continuity, availability, protectedness, and support come through in Ms. H.'s description of her relationship with two key caregivers.

3. **Caregiving transactions have a psychotherapeutic dimension.** Caregivers at the bedside are usually not trained mental health professionals. Such bedside care is ordinarily provided to restore bodily function to an optimal degree. The methods used are technical and focused on technique. Yet Ms. H. gives a clear message in her vignette that the care was psychologically healing as well as physiologically restorative. She says of her nurse, "[She saved] my sanity . . . she treated me as if nothing was wrong with me; she was rough and humorous. . . ." This particular nurse made Ms. H. feel "normal" psychologically, even as her body was far from normal. Such skill has psychotherapeutic dimensions that are clearly recalled 40 years later. For Ms. H. her *body* healed over a period of several months. The *psychological* healing is a different matter and may never be fully completed. Yet the care she initially received made an important psychological contribution to her current self concept.

4. **Caregivers are nonjudgmental in their tolerance of the suffering of others. Empathy is the tool that forms the basis of good care.** Ms. H. recalls that while the interns removed the bandages, her physician would stand at the head of the bed and instruct her to cry out and scream. "Of course, I couldn't, but it made me feel brave, especially when he said, 'I know what you're going through.'" The phrase Ms. H. can recall her surgeon making almost a half century later is, "I know what you're going through." This particular care-

giver did not excuse himself during the painful dressing changes, but provided the emotional support for Ms. H. even as the interns were carrying out the strictly medical activities. (This is an interesting example of psychomedical teamwork.) No information is available on how the physician himself coped with this daily routine of pain, but one can speculate that this was not a pleasant experience for either patient or caregiver. One can surmise that feeling some of the pain himself was a necessary prelude to the empathic response this surgeon made to Ms. H.

Tolerating the suffering of others in a nonjudgmental and empathic fashion is central to good caregiving. Emphasized throughout this work is the notion that caregivers neither "attack" their patients out of frustration nor abandon them out of a sense of despair. While one may *feel* each of these emotions about any particular patient strongly, one's stance is to remain available in the face of these pressures. This is easier said than done. Part of the job is to absorb some of the pain of this work without "acting out" this pain. One of the initial reviewers of the manuscript of this monograph pointed out that considerable pain seemed present in the caregivers themselves as well as in the patients described here. Giving care to those who suffer means in some fashion to share in that suffering. Entering into the suffering of others carries no guarantees that one's efforts will receive recognition or acknowledgment. The sense of being helped may breed resentment instead of gratitude. This in itself can contribute to the pain of caregiving.

5. **Self-reflection and self-understanding are essential to good caregiving.** Unfortunately we could not interview Ms. H.'s caregivers directly, but Ms. H. herself provides a good example of the self-reflective stance espoused in this work. She carefully balances the distress and disfigurement she experienced with the quality of the care she received. For example, she says of her surgeon, "He made all the pain endurable because he cared so much." Ms. H. gives the impression that while her life has been a struggle since her injury, it is a struggle that was balanced by caregiving responses that made it at least tolerable.

Throughout our discussions in this report we have emphasized the ability to step back from the experiences of caregiving in order to gain some perspective. Through team meetings, retreats, vacations, and informal discussions, the importance of a reflective stance toward this work has been emphasized. To neglect this aspect of our effort is to risk losing "touch" with our patients and with ourselves. Care can become rote and perfunctory, in which case the caregiver loses the opportunity to grow and learn from the caregiving experience.

6. **Caregivers can bring about positive change through their involvement.** Ms. H.'s nurse was affectionately described as "rough and humorous." One senses an inner strength in this woman that directly contributed to Ms. H.'s recovery from her burns. Despite the enormity of our caregiving goals, still we can be optimistic about change. We can always make things a bit better; if not in large ways, then in small ways; if not in our patient, then at least in ourselves. The transactions the caregiver has with a person with a physical impairment implicitly contain within them the promise of hope and the potential for change in both individuals so engaged.

Our committee has attempted to describe the transactions that occur between a professional caregiver and a person with a life-altering, appearance-altering physical impairment. Emphasized throughout has been the rich, complex subjective dimension of these transactions. This dimension included the building of a relationship with the patient, the recognition and management of the feelings generated in the caregiver by that relationship, and ways to cope with the vicissitudes and/or challenges inherent in this experience. Not only have the risks, the pain, and the frustration of this activity been described, but the satisfactions and fulfillment inherent in caregiving have been spelled out as well.

The historical and societal components of care have been alluded to as they impinge on bedside transactions between caregiver and patient. Traditional caregiver-patient tensions and social stigma make their contributions to these processes. The caregiver-patient arena has been traced from its more traditional "bedside" setting within the hospital/rehabilitation center to the community, family, and workplace. Concomitant with this change comes a shift from "professional" caregiving to more informal systems of care in the home and neighborhood. The well-structured system of care in the hospital shifts to a kaleidoscopic panoply of services in the community, and this transition has not escaped our attention.

We leave the complex Judeo-Christian value systems, and the spiritual/aesthetic principles undergirding this caregiving role, for others to articulate. As we close, however, we are reminded of the deep ethical basis on which our activities rest by a quotation from Christopher Nolan. This young man has been imprisoned by his mute and paralyzed body since birth. He found his voice with the aid of a typing stick attached to his head. The excerpt below (in which he refers to himself as "Joseph") about his caregivers (referred to as teachers) was taken from his book *Under the Eye of the Clock*:

> Such were Joseph's teachers and such their imagination that the mute boy became constantly amazed at the almost telepathic degree of

certainty with which they read his facial expression, eye movements and body language. Many a good laugh was had by teacher and pupil as they deciphered his code. It was at moments such as these that Joseph recognized the face of God in human form. It glimmered in their kindness to him, it glowed in their keenness, it hinted in their caring, indeed it caressed in their gaze. (Nolan 1987, p. 11)

# References

Apt AF: Alt-Garrison History of Pediatrics. Philadelphia, PA, WB Saunders, 1965

Asch A, Rousso H: Therapists with disabilities: theoretical and clinical issues. Psychiatry 48:1–12, 1985

Basch M: Doing Psychotherapy. New York, Basic Books, 1980

Basch M: Understanding Psychotherapy. New York, Basic Books, 1988

Berkowitz M: Disincentives and the rehabilitation of disabled persons, in Annual Review of Rehabilitation, Vol 2. Edited by Pan EL, Backer TE, Vask CL. New York, Springer, 1981, pp 40–57

Bohr N: Das Quantenysostulat and Die nuere entwickleng der Aposmistik. Natwevissin-schaften 16:245, 1928

Book HE: Empathy: misconceptions and misuses in psychotherapy. Am J Psychiatry 145:420–425, 1988

Bowe F: Rehabilitating America: Barriers to Disabled People. New York, Harper & Row, 1980

Bracken MB, Bernstein M: Adaptation to and coping with disability one year after spinal cord injury: an epidemiological study. Social Psychiatry 15:33–41, 1980

Bray GP: Family adaptation to chronic illness, in Rehabilitation Psychology Desk Reference. Edited by Kaplan B. Rockville, MD, Aspen, 1987, pp 171–183

Burns RP: The Self Concept. London, Longman, 1975

Castelnuovo-Tedesco P: Psychological consequences of physical defects and trauma, in Emotional Rehabilitation of Physical Trauma and Disability. Edited by Hunt D. New York, Spectrum, 1984, pp 25–34

Caywood TA: A quadriplegic young man looks at treatment. Journal of Rehabilitation 49(6):22–25, 1974

Chambers R: Victim invicta in stigma, in Stigma: The Experience of Disability. Edited by Hunt P. London, Geoffrey Chapman, 1966, pp 18–28

Cogswell BE: Self-socialization: readjustment of paraplegics in the community. Journal of Rehabilitation 34:11–13, 1968

Coles R: The Call of Stories. New York, Houghton-Mifflin, 1989

Cumming J, Cumming E: Ego and Milieu. New York, Atherton Press, 1963

Darling RB: Social and professional reactions to congenital handicaps, in Children Who Are Different. Edited by Darling RB, Darling EF. St Louis, MO, CV Mosby, 1982, pp 31–48

Davis F: Deviance disavowal: the management of strained interactions in the visibly handicapped, in The Other Side. Edited by Becker HS. New York, Free Press, 1964, pp 118–137

DeGuire L: The wounded healer. Unpublished doctoral dissertation, University of Pennsylvania, Philadelphia, PA, 1990

DeLisa JA, Martin GM, Currie DM: Rehabilitation medicine: past, present and future, in Rehabilitation Medicine: Principles and Practice. Edited by DeLisa JA. Philadelphia, PA, JB Lippincott, 1988, pp 1–24

DeLoach C, Green BG: Adjustment to Severe Physical Disability: A Metamorphosis. New York, McGraw-Hill, 1981

Emde RN, Harmon RJ, Good W: Depressive feelings in children: a transactional model for research, in Depression in Young People. Edited by Rutter M, Izard C, Read P. New York, Guilford, 1986, pp 135–160

Erikson E: A schedule of virtues, in Insight and Responsibility. New York, WW Norton, 1964

Erikson E: Life History and the Historical Moment. New York, WW Norton, 1975

Feagin JR: Subordinating the Poor: Welfare and American Beliefs. Englewood Cliffs, NJ, Prentice-Hall, 1975

Featherstone H: A Difference in the Family: Life With a Disabled Child. New York, Basic Books, 1980

Gans JS: Hate in the rehabilitation setting. Arch Phys Med Rehabil 64:176–186, 1983

Giamatti AB: Yale Magazine, Vol 44, December 1989, p 14

Gliedman J, Roth W: The Unexpected Minority: Handicapped Children in America. New York, Harcourt Brace Jovanovich, 1980

Goffman E: Asylums: Essays on the Social Situation of Mental Patients and Other Inmates. Garden City, NY, Doubleday, 1961

Goffman E: Stigma: Notes on the Management of Spoiled Identity. Englewood Cliffs, NJ, Prentice-Hall, 1963

Goldman G: Environmental barriers to sociocultural integration: the insider's perspective. Rehabilitation Literature 39:185–189, 1978

Graves JE: Taking care of the hateful patient. N Engl J Med 298:883–887, 1978

Grinker RR: Biomedical education as a system. Arch Gen Psychiatry 24:291–298, 1971

Group for the Advancement of Psychiatry: Psychiatric Consultation in Mental Retardation. GAP Report No 104. New York, Group for the Advancement of Psychiatry, 1979

Gunther MS: The threatened staff: a psychoanalytic contribution to medical psychology. Compr Psychiatry 18:385–394, 1977

Gunther MS: The pathology of psychiatric consultations: a different view. Compr Psychiatry 20:187–198, 1979

Hahn H: The social component of sexuality and disability: some problems and proposals. Sexuality and Disability 4(4):220–233, 1981

Hahn H: Paternalism and public policy. Society 20(3):36–46, 1983

Hamburg DA, Adams JE: A perspective on coping behavior. Arch Gen Psychiatry 17:277–284, 1967

Harter S, Buddin BJ: Children's understanding of the simultaneity of two emotions: a five-stage developmental acquisition sequence. Developmental Psychology 23:388–399, 1987

Heisenberg W: Uber den anschaulichen Inhalt der quanten Theorictischen: "Kimematik und Merchanic." Zeitschrift für Physik 43:172, 1927

Hoffter J: The changeling: history and psychodynamics of attributes to handicapped children in European folklore. J Hist Behav Sci 4:55–61, 1968

Horowitz M: Stress Response Syndromes. New York, Jason Aronson, 1976

Hull JM: Touching the Rock: An Experience of Blindness. New York, Pantheon, 1991

Ittelson WH: Perceptions and transactional psychology, in Psychology: A Study of a Science. Edited by Koch S. New York, McGraw-Hill, 1962, pp 660–704

Keith RA: Observations in the Rehabilitation Hospital: Twenty Years of Research. Arch Phys Med Rehabil 69:625–631, 1988

Kerr N: Staff expectations for disabled persons: helpful or harmful? in Social and Psychological Aspects of Disability. Edited by Stubbins J. Baltimore, MD, University Park Press, 1977, pp 47–54

Kleck R: Emotional arousal in interactions with stigmatized persons. Psychol Rep 19:1226, 1966

Kohut H: Analysis of the Self. New York, International Universities Press, 1971

Kohut H: The Restoration of the Self. New York, International Universities Press, 1977

Krueger DW: An Overview in Emotional Rehabilitation of Physical Trauma and Disability. New York, Spectrum, 1984, pp 3–12

Lawn B: Experiences of a paraplegic psychiatry resident on an inpatient psychiatric unit. Am J Psychiatry 146:771–774, 1989

Lazarus RS, Folkman S: Stress, Appraisal and Coping. New York, Springer, 1984

Lenz R, Chaves B: Becoming active partners: a couple's perspective, in Sexuality and Physical Disability: Personal Perspectives. Edited by Bullard DG, Knight SE. St Louis, MO, CV Mosby, 1981, pp 65–67

Lewiston NJ, Conley J, Blessing-Moore J: Measurement of hypothetical burnout in cystic fibrosis caregivers. Acta Paediatr Scand 70:935–939, 1981

Maus-Clum N, Ryan M: Brain injury and the family. Journal of Neurosurgical Nursing 13:165–169, 1981

Meyer E, Mendelson J: Psychiatric consultation with patients on medical and surgical wards: patterns and processes. Psychiatry 24:197–220, 1961

Meyerson R: Family and parent group therapy, in The Family With a Handicapped Child. Edited by Seligman M. New York, Grune & Stratton, 1983, pp 285–308

Miller J: The Body in Question. New York, Vantage Press, 1978

Mullins LL: Hate revisited: power, envy, and greed in the rehabilitation setting. Arch Phys Med Rehabil 70:740–744, 1989

Newman J: Handicapped persons and their families: philosophical, historical and legislative perspectives, in The Family With a Handicapped Child. Edited by Seligman M. New York, Grune & Stratton, 1983, pp 3–26

Niederland WG: Narcissistic ego impairment in patients with early physical malformations. Psychoanal Study Child 20:518–534, 1965

Nolan C: Under the Eye of the Clock. New York, St Martin's Press, 1987

Nussbaum K: Subjective elements in rehabilitation, in Emotional Rehabilitation of Physical Trauma and Disability. Edited by Kruger DW. New York, Spectrum, 1984, pp 183–194

Palmer S, Conn L, Sibens AA, et al: Psychosocial services in rehabilitation medicine: an interdisciplinary approach. Arch Phys Med Rehabil 66:690–692, 1985

Pasnau RO: Consultation-Liaison Psychiatry. New York, Grune & Stratton, 1975

Perrin JM, MacLean WE: Children with chronic illness. Pediatr Clin North Am 35:1325–1337, 1988

Purtillo RB: Ethical issues in teamwork: the context of rehabilitation. Arch Phys Med Rehabil 69:318–322, 1988

Rothberg JJ: The interdisciplinary process: is it a chimera for clinical practice and for the ACRM? Arch Phys Med Rehabil 66:343–347, 1985

Rusk HA: Rehabilitation Medicine. St Louis, MO, CV Mosby, 1977

Sacks O: A Leg to Stand On. New York, Harper & Row, 1984

Safilios-Rothchild C: The Sociology and Social Psychology of Disability and Rehabilitation. New York, Random House, 1970

Sameroff AJ, Chandler M: Reproductive risk and the continuum of caretaking casualty, in Review of Child Development Research, Vol 4. Edited by Horowitz F. Chicago, IL, University of Chicago Press, 1975, pp 187–244

Schilder P: The Image and Appearance of the Human Body. New York, International Universities Press, 1950

Schwab JJ: Psychiatric illness in medical patients: why it goes undiagnosed. Psychosomatics 23:221–229, 1982

Smith D: Spinal cord injury, in Sexuality and Physical Disability: Personal Perspectives. Edited by Bullard DG, Knight SE. St Louis, MO, CV Mosby, 1981, pp 12–25

Smith JK, Plimpton G: New York Times, June 11, 1989, p 46

Smith RT, Behart AJ: Social policy issues in invalidity programs: crossnational perspectives, in Cross-National Rehabilitation Policies: A Sociological Perspective. Edited by Albrecht GL. Beverly Hills, CA, Sage, 1981

Stotland NL, Garrick TR: Manual of Psychiatric Consultation. Washington, DC, American Psychiatric Press, 1990

Stubbins J: Stress and disability, in Social and Psychological Aspects of Disability. Edited by Stubbins J. Baltimore, MD, University Park Press, 1977, pp 475–480

Stuber ML, Sullivan G, Kennon TL, et al: Group therapy for chronic medical illnesses: a multi-diagnosis group. Gen Hosp Psychiatry 10:360–366, 1988

Tarnow JD: Pediatric and adolescent patients in rehabilitation, in Emotional Rehabilitation of Physical Trauma and Disability. Edited by Krueger DW. New York, Spectrum, 1984, pp 63–78

Thomas D: The Experience of Handicap. London, Methuen, 1982

Turner RJ, Beiser M: Major depression and depressive symptomatology among the physically disabled. J Nerv Ment Dis 178:343–350, 1990

Urbach JR, Culbert JP: Head-injured children and their parents: psychosocial consequences of a traumatic syndrome. Psychosomatics 32:24–33, 1991

Voight MA: Courage: The Story of Courage Center. Golden Valley, MN, Courage Center, 1989

Winnicott DW: Transitional objects and transitional phenomena, in Collected Papers. New York, Tavistock/Barnes & Noble, 1958

Worthington ME: Personal space as a function of stigma effect, in Social and Psychological Aspects of Disability. Edited by Stubbins J. Baltimore, MD, University Park Press, 1977, pp 287–291

# GAP Committees and Membership

## Committee on Adolescence

Warren J. Gadpaille, Denver, CO, *Chairperson*
Hector R. Bird, New York, NY
Ian A. Canino, New York, NY
Michael G. Kalogerakis, New York, NY
Paulina F. Kernberg, New York, NY
Clarice J. Kestenbaum, New York, NY
Richard C. Marohn, Chicago, IL
Silvio J. Onesti, Jr., Belmont, MA

## Committee on Aging

Gene D. Cohen, Washington, DC, *Chairperson*
Karen Blank, West Hartford, CT
Eric D. Caine, Rochester, NY
Charles M. Gaitz, Houston, TX
Gary Gottlieb, Philadelphia, PA
Ira R. Katz, Philadelphia, PA
Andrew F. Leuchter, Los Angeles, CA
Gabe J. Maletta, Minneapolis, MN
Richard A. Margolin, Nashville, TN
Kenneth M. Sakauye, New Orleans, LA
Charles A. Shamoian, Larchmont, NY
F. Conyers Thompson, Jr., Atlanta, GA

## Committee on Alcoholism and the Addictions

Joseph Westermeyer, Minneapolis, MN, *Chairperson*
Margaret H. Bean-Bayog, Lexington, MA
Susan J. Blumenthal, Washington, DC
Richard J. Frances, Newark, NJ
Marc Galanter, New York, NY
Earl A. Loomis, Jr., Augusta, GA
Sheldon I. Miller, Chicago, IL

Edgar P. Nace, Dallas, TX
Peter Steinglass, Washington, DC
John S. Tamerin, Greenwich, CT

## Committee on Child Psychiatry

Peter E. Tanguay, Los Angeles, CA, *Chairperson*
James M. Bell, Canaan, NY
Mark Blotcky, Dallas, TX
Harlow Donald Dunton, New York, NY
Joseph Fischhoff, Detroit, MI
Joseph M. Green, Madison, WI
John F. McDermott, Jr., Honolulu, HI
David A. Mrazek, Denver, CO
Cynthia R. Pfeffer, White Plains, NY
John Schowalter, New Haven, CT
Theodore Shapiro, New York, NY
Leonore Terr, San Francisco, CA

## Committee on College Students

Earle Silber, Chevy Chase, MD, *Chairperson*
Robert L. Arnstein, Hamden, CT
Varda Backus, La Jolla, CA
Harrison P. Eddy, New York, NY
Myron B. Liptzin, Chapel Hill, NC
Malkah Tolpin Notman, Brookline, MA
Gloria C. Onque, Pittsburgh, PA
Elizabeth Aub Reid, Cambridge, MA
Lorraine D. Siggins, New Haven, CT
Tom G. Stauffer, White Plains, NY

## Committee on Cultural Psychiatry

Ezra Griffith, New Haven, CT, *Chairperson*
Edward Foulks, New Orleans, LA
Pedro Ruiz, Houston, TX
Ronald Wintrob, Providence, RI
Joe Yamamoto, Los Angeles, CA

## Committee on the Family

Herta A. Guttman, Montreal, PQ, *Chairperson*
W. Robert Beavers, Dallas, TX

Ellen M. Berman, Merion, PA
Ira D. Glick, New York, NY
Frederick Gottlieb, Los Angeles, CA
Henry U. Grunebaum, Cambridge, MA
Judith Landau-Stanton, Rochester, NY
Ann L. Price, Avon, CT
Lyman C. Wynne, Rochester, NY

## Committee on Government Policy

Roger Peele, Washington, DC, *Chairperson*
Thomas L. Clannon, San Francisco, CA
Naomi Heller, Washington, DC
John P. D. Shemo, Charlottesville, VA
William W. Van Stone, Washington, DC

## Committee on Handicaps

William H. Sack, Portland, OR, *Chairperson*
Norman R. Bernstein, Cambridge, MA
Meyer S. Gunther, Wilmette, IL
Bryan King, Los Angeles, CA
Robert Nesheim, Duluth, MN
Betty J. Pfefferbaum, Norman, OK
William A. Sonis, Philadelphia, PA
Margaret L. Stuber, Los Angeles, CA
George Tarjan, Los Angeles, CA
Thomas G. Webster, Washington, DC
Henry H. Work, Bethesda, MD

## Committee on Human Sexuality

Bertram H. Schaffner, New York, NY, *Chairperson*
Paul L. Adams, Galveston, TX
Debra Carter, Farmington, NM
Richard Friedman, New York, NY
Peggy Hanley-Hackenbruck, Portland, OR
Johanna A. Hoffman, Scottsdale, AZ
Joan A. Lang, Galveston, TX
Stuart E. Nichols, New York, NY
Harris B. Peck, New Rochelle, NY
Terry S. Stein, East Lansing, MI

## Committee on International Relations

Vamik D. Volkan, Charlottesville, VA, *Chairperson*
Robert M. Dorn, El Macero, CA
John S. Kafka, Washington, DC
Otto F. Kernberg, White Plains, NY
Roy W. Menninger, Topeka, KS
Peter A. Olsson, Houston, TX
Rita R. Rogers, Palos Verdes Estates, CA
Stephen B. Shanfield, San Antonio, TX

## Committee on Medical Education

Steven L. Dubovsky, Denver, CO, *Chairperson*
Leah Dickstein, Louisville, KY
Saul I. Harrison, Torrance, CA
David R. Hawkins, Chicago, IL
Jerry Kay, Dayton, OH
Harold I. Lief, Philadelphia, PA
Carol C. Nadelson, Boston, MA
Carolyn B. Robinowitz, Washington, DC
Stephen C. Scheiber, Deerfield, IL
Sidney L. Werkman, Washington, DC

## Committee on Mental Health Services

W. Walter Menninger, Topeka, KS, *Chairperson*
Mary Jane England, Roseland, NJ
Robert O. Friedel, Richmond, VA
John M. Hamilton, Columbia, MD
Jose Maria Santiago, Tucson, AZ
Steven S. Sharfstein, Baltimore, MD
George F. Wilson, Somerville, NJ
Jack A. Wolford, Pittsburgh, PA

## Committee on Planning and Communications

Robert W. Gibson, Towson, MD, *Chairperson*
Allan Beigel, Tucson, AZ
Doyle I. Carson, Dallas, TX
Paul J. Fink, Philadelphia, PA
Robert S. Garber, Longboat Key, FL
Richard K. Goodstein, Belle Mead, NJ
Harvey L. Ruben, New Haven, CT

Melvin Sabshin, Washington, DC
Michael R. Zales, Quechee, VT

## Committee on Preventive Psychiatry

Naomi Rae-Grant, London, ON, *Chairperson*
Viola W. Bernard, New York, NY
Stephen Fleck, New Haven, CT
Brian J. McConville, Cincinnati, OH
David R. Offord, Hamilton, Ont.
Morton M. Silverman, Chicago, IL
Warren T. Vaughan, Jr., Portola Valley, CA
Ann Marie Wolf-Schatz, Conshohocken, PA

## Committee on Psychiatry and the Community

H. Richard Lamb, Los Angeles, CA, *Chairperson*
C. Knight Aldrich, Charlottesville, VA
Stephen Goldfinger, Boston, MA
David G. Greenfield, Guilford, CT
Kenneth Minkoff, Woburn, MA
John C. Nemiah, Hanover, NH
John J. Schwab, Louisville, KY
Allan Tasman, Louisville, KY
Charles B. Wilkinson, Kansas City, MO

## Committee on Psychiatry and the Law

Joseph Satten, San Francisco, CA, *Chairperson*
J. Richard Ciccone, Rochester, NY
Carl P. Malmquist, Minneapolis, MN
Jeffrey Metzner, Denver, CO
Herbert C. Modlin, Topeka, KS
Jonas R. Rappeport, Baltimore, MD
Phillip J. Resnick, Cleveland, OH
Robert I. Simon, Bethesda, MD
William D. Weitzel, Lexington, KY

## Committee on Psychiatry and Religion

Richard C. Lewis, New Haven, CT, *Chairperson*
Naleen N. Andrade, Honolulu, HI
Keith G. Meador, Nashville, TN
Abigail R. Ostow, Belmont, MA

## Committee on Research

Zebulon Taintor, New York, NY, *Chairperson*
Robert Cancro, New York, NY
John H. Greist, Madison, WI
Jerry M. Lewis, Dallas, TX
John G. Looney, Durham, NC
Sidney Malitz, New York, NY

## Committee on Social Issues

Ian E. Alger, New York, NY, *Chairperson*
William R. Beardslee, Waban, MA
Roderic Gorney, Los Angeles, CA
Martha J. Kirkpatrick, Los Angeles, CA
Perry Ottenberg, Philadelphia, PA
Kendon W. Smith, Pearl River, NY

## Committee on Therapeutic Care

William W. Richards, Anchorage, AK, *Chairperson*
Bernard Bandler, Cambridge, MA
Thomas E. Curtis, Chapel Hill, NC
Donald C. Fidler, Morgantown, WV
Donald W. Hammersley, Washington, DC
William B. Hunter, III, Albuquerque, NM
Roberto L. Jimenez, San Antonio, TX
Milton Kramer, Cincinnati, OH
John Lipkin, Perry Point, MA
Theodore Nadelson, Jamaica Plain, MA

## Committee on Therapy

Jules R. Bemporad, White Plains, NY, *Chairperson*
Gerald Adler, Boston, MA
Eugene B. Feigelson, Brooklyn, NY
Robert Michels, New York, NY
Andrew P. Morrison, Cambridge, MA
William C. Offenkrantz, Scottsdale, AZ
Allan D. Rosenblatt, La Jolla, CA

## GINSBURG FELLOWS

Michael R. Arambula, Chicago, IL *(Committee on Government Policy)*

B. James Bennett, Dallas, TX *(Committee on Adolescence)*

Deborah L. Cabaniss, New York, NY *(Committee on Medical Education)*

Laura J. Dalheim, Barrington, RI *(Committee on Therapeutic Care)*

Alex R. Demac, New Haven, CT *(Committee on Public Education)*

Hinda F. Dubin, Baltimore, MD *(Committee on Psychiatry and Religion)*

James R. Dumerauf, Waukesha, WI *(Committee on Handicaps)*

Denise M. Heebink, New York, NY *(Committee on International Relations)*

Patricia L. Hough, Augusta, GA *(Committee on Social Issues)*

Jonathan House, New York, NY *(Committee on Therapy)*

David J. Kapley, Chapel Hill, NC *(Committee on Psychiatry and the Law)*

Shitij Kapur, Pittsburgh, PA *(Committee on Psychopathology)*

Debra F. Kirsch, Houston, TX *(Committee on Alcoholism and the Addictions)*

Laura W. Lane, Albuquerque, NM *(Committee on Preventive Psychiatry)*

Constantine G. Lyketsos, Baltimore, MD *(Committee on Research)*

Elizabeth A. Murphy, Boston, MA *(Committee on Cultural Psychiatry)*

Michel Paradis, Montreal, PQ *(Committee on Psychiatry in Industry)*

Linda M. Peterson, Owings Mills, MD *(Committee on Psychiatry and the Community)*

Anthony Poehailos, Charlottesville, VA *(Committee on Child Psychiatry)*

Rachel G. Seidel, Belmont, MA *(Committee on Planning and Communications)*

Rita A. Shaughnessy, Oak Park, IL *(Committee on Mental Health Services)*

Joseph A. Shrand, West Simsbury, CT *(Committee on the Family)*

Grace C. Vigilante, New Orleans, LA *(Committee on College Students)*

Susan L. Warren, Somerville, MA *(Committee on Aging)*

Gwen L. Zornberg, Belmont, MA *(Committee on Human Sexuality)*

## Contributing Members

Gene Abroms, Ardmore, PA
Carlos C. Alden, Jr., Buffalo, NY
Kenneth Z. Altshuler, Dallas, TX
Francis F. Barnes, Washington, DC
Spencer Bayles, Houston, TX
C. Christian Beels, New York, NY
Elissa P. Benedek, Ann Arbor, MI
Sidney Berman, Washington, DC
Renee L. Binder, San Francisco, CA
H. Keith H. Brodie, Durham, NC
Charles M. Bryant, San Francisco, CA
Ewald W. Busse, Durham, NC
Robert N. Butler, New York, NY
Eugene M. Caffey, Jr., Bowie, MD
Robert J. Campbell, New York, NY
James P. Cattell, San Diego, CA
Ian L.W. Clancey, Maitland, ON
Sanford I. Cohen, Coral Gables, FL
Lee Combrinck-Graham, Evanston, IL
Charles M. Culver, Hanover, NH
Robert E. Drake, Hanover, NH
James S. Eaton, Jr., Washington, DC
Lloyd C. Elam, Nashville, TN
Joseph T. English, New York, NY
Sherman C. Feinstein, Highland Park, IL
Archie R. Foley, New York, NY
Sidney Furst, Bronx, NY
Henry J. Gault, Highland Park, IL
Judith H. Gold, Halifax, NS
Alexander Gralnick, Port Chester, NY
Milton Greenblatt, Sylmar, CA
Lawrence F. Greenleigh, Los Angeles, CA
Stanley I. Greenspan, Bethesda, MD
Jon E. Gudeman, Milwaukee, WI
Stanley Hammons, Lexington, KY
William Hetznecker, Merion Station, PA
J. Cotter Hirschberg, Topeka, KS
Johanna A. Hoffman, Scottsdale, AZ
Jay Katz, New Haven, CT
Edward J. Khantzian, Haverhill, MA
James A. Knight, New Orleans, LA

Othilda M. Krug, Cincinnati, OH
Anthony F. Lehman, Baltimore, MD
Alan I. Levenson, Tucson, AZ
Ruth W. Lidz, Woodbridge, CT
Orlando B. Lightfoot, Boston, MA
Norman L. Loux, Sellersville, PA
Albert J. Lubin, Woodside, CA
John Mack, Chestnut Hill, MA
John A. MacLeod, Cincinnati, OH
Charles A. Malone, Barrington, RI
Peter A. Martin, Lake Orion, MI
Ake Mattsson, Charlottesville, VA
Alan A. McLean, Gig Harbor, WA
David Mendell, Houston, TX
Mary E. Mercer, Nyack, NY
Derek Miller, Chicago, IL
Steven M. Mirin, Belmont, MA
Richard D. Morrill, Boston, MA
Robert J. Nathan, Philadelphia, PA
Joseph D. Noshpitz, Washington, DC
Mortimer Ostow, Bronx, NY
Bernard L. Pacella, New York, NY
Herbert Pardes, New York, NY
Norman L. Paul, Lexington, MA
Marvin E. Perkins, Salem, VA
George H. Pollock, Chicago, IL
Becky Potter, Tucson, AZ
David N. Ratnavale, Bethesda, MD
Richard E. Renneker, Pacific Palisades, CA
W. Donald Ross, Cincinnati, OH
Loren Roth, Pittsburgh, PA
Donald J. Scherl, Brooklyn, NY
Charles Shagass, Philadelphia, PA
Miles F. Shore, Boston, MA
Albert J. Silverman, Ann Arbor, MI
Benson R. Snyder, Cambridge, MA
David A. Soskis, Bala Cynwyd, PA
Jeffrey L. Speller, Cambridge, MA
Jeanne Spurlock, Washington, DC
Brandt F. Steele, Denver, CO
Alan A. Stone, Cambridge, MA
Perry C. Talkington, Dallas, TX
John Talbott, Baltimore, MD

Bryce Templeton, Philadelphia, PA
Prescott W. Thompson, Portland, OR
John A. Turner, San Francisco, CA
Gene L. Usdin, New Orleans, LA
Kenneth N. Vogtsberger, San Antonio, TX
Andrew S. Watson, Ann Arbor, MI
Joseph B. Wheelwright, Kentfield, CA
Robert L. Williams, Houston, TX
Paul Tyler Wilson, Bethesda, MD
Sherwyn M. Woods, Los Angeles, CA
Kent A. Zimmerman, Menlo Park, CA
Howard Zonana, New Haven, CT

## Life Members

C. Knight Aldrich, Charlottesville, VA
Robert L. Arnstein, Hamden, CT
Bernard Bandler, Cambridge, MA
Walter E. Barton, Hartland, VT
Viola W. Bernard, New York, NY
Henry W. Brosin, Tucson, AZ
John Donnelly, Hartford, CT
Merrill T. Eaton, Omaha, NE
O. Spurgeon English, Narberth, PA
Stephen Fleck, New Haven, CT
Jerome Frank, Baltimore, MD
Robert S. Garber, Longboat Key, FL
Robert I. Gibson, Towson, MD
Margaret M. Lawrence, Pomona, NY
Jerry M. Lewis, Dallas, TX
Harold I. Lief, Philadelphia, PA
Judd Marmor, Los Angeles, CA
Herbert C. Modlin, Topeka, KS
John C. Nemiah, Hanover, NH
William C. Offenkrantz, Scottsdale, AZ
Mabel Ross, Sun City, AZ
Julius Schreiber, Washington, DC
Robert E. Switzer, Dunn Loring, VA
Jack A. Wolford, Pittsburgh, PA
Henry H. Work, Bethesda, MD

## BOARD OF DIRECTORS

## Officers

*President*
Allan Beigel
P.O. Box 43460
Tucson, AZ   85733

*President-Elect*
Charles Wilkinson
1232 W. 64th Terrace
Kansas City, MO   64113

*Secretary*
Doyle I. Carson
Timberlawn Psychiatric Hospital
P.O. Box 151489
Dallas, TX   75315-1489

*Treasurer*
Jack W. Bonner, III
The Oaks Treatment Center
1407 West Stassney Lane
Austin, TX   78745

*Board Members*
Malkah Notman
Naomi Rae-Grant
Stephen Scheiber
Joe Yamamoto

*Past Presidents*
*William C. Menninger 1946–51
Jack R. Ewalt 1951–53
Walter E. Barton 1953–55
*Sol W. Ginsburg 1955–57
*Dana L. Farnsworth 1957–59
*Marion E. Kenworthy 1959–61

---

*Deceased.

Henry W. Brosin 1961–63
*Leo H. Bartemeier 1963–65
Robert S. Garber 1965–67
Herbert C. Modlin 1967–69
John Donnelly 1969–71
George Tarjan 1971–73
Judd Marmor 1973–75
John C. Nemiah 1975–77
Jack A. Wolford 1977–79
Robert W. Gibson 1979–81
*Jack Weinberg 1981–82
Henry H. Work 1982–85
Michael R. Zales 1985–87
Jerry M. Lewis 1987–89
Carolyn B. Robinowitz 1989–91

## PUBLICATIONS BOARD

*Chairperson*
C. Knight Aldrich
Health Sciences Center
Box 414
Charlottesville, VA 22908

Robert L. Arnstein
Mark Blotcky
Judith H. Gold
Ezra Griffith
Steve Katz
Milton Kramer
W. Walter Menninger
Robert A. Solow

*Consultants* .
John C. Nemiah
Henry H. Work

*Ex-Officio*
Allan Beigel
Carolyn B. Robinowitz

---

*Deceased.

## CONTRIBUTORS

Abbott Laboratories
American Charitable Fund
Dr. and Mrs. Richard Aron
Mr. Robert C. Baker
Bristol-Myers Squibb Co.
Maurice Falk Medical Fund
Mrs. Carol Gold
Edith F. Goldensohn
Grove Foundation, Inc.
Miss Gayle Groves
Ittleson Foundation, Inc.
Mr. Barry Jacobson
Mrs. Allan H. Kalmus
Marion E. Kenworthy–Sarah H. Swift Foundation, Inc.
Mr. Larry Korman
McNeil Pharmaceutical
Murel Foundation
Phillips Foundation
Sandoz Corporation
Smith Kline Beckman Corporation
Tappanz Foundation, Inc.
The Upjohn Company
van Ameringen Foundation, Inc.
Wyeth-Ayerst Laboratories
Mr. and Mrs. William A. Zales

# Index